"As someone who's no stranger to both the kitchen and the occasional puff, I can't say enough good things about Vanessa Lavorato's *How to Eat Weed & Have a Good Time*. This book isn't just about cooking with cannabis, it's about elevating your entire experience. Vanessa breaks down the science and the art of it all, making it feel like you're cooking alongside a friend who just happens to be a total expert. If you love good food and a good high, this is the cookbook you didn't know you needed."

—TESS SINATRO, @Lamb_Chop97

"Books like this are necessary! Especially coming from someone like Vanessa, who has been passionate about educating people on how to cook with cannabis for many years. She is one of the most knowledgeable people I know in the field. It's a must-read!"

—B-REAL, Cypress Hill

"*How to Eat Wee[d]* *Time* is the ultim[ate] on getting bake[d] Vanessa explai[ns] [everything from] the science of getting high to how and where you can physically buy weed to, obviously, how to cook with it like a true expert. She spares no details, and while I've never cooked with weed myself, this is where I'd want to learn."

—HENRY LAPORTE, author of *Salt Hank*

"If there is anyone that I'm gonna trust to take me on a fun, weed-filled journey, it's Vanessa. Not only is her book educational and filled with exciting, clever recipes that you'll want to cook over and over but the photography is gorgeous and the recipes are dosed in a way that allows you to control your cannabis intake and consume enough weed to get you stoned but also eat as much of the dish as you'd like. And believe me, you're going to want to make everything in this cookbook."

—FARIDEH SADEGHIN, cookbook author and content creator

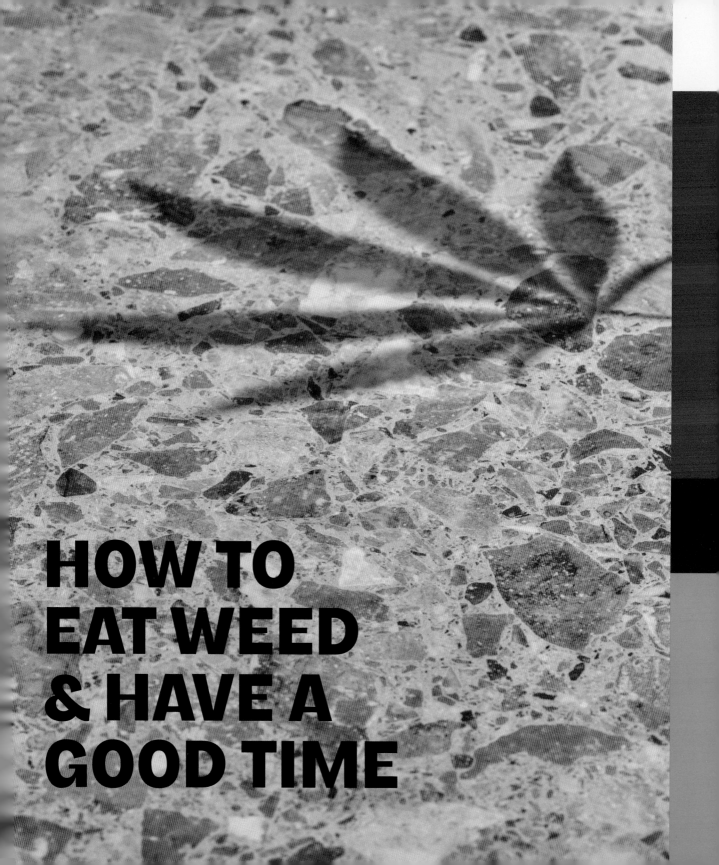

HOW TO
EAT WEED
& HAVE A
GOOD TIME

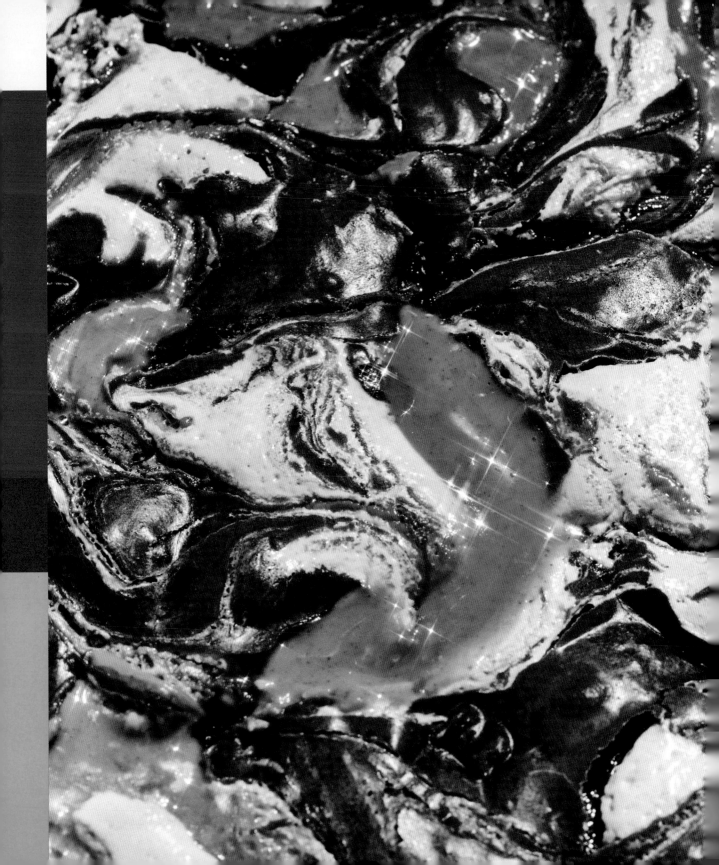

HOW TO EAT WEED & HAVE A GOOD TIME

A CANNABIS COOKBOOK

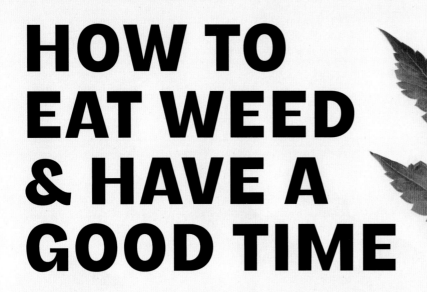

VANESSA LAVORATO

PHOTOGRAPHY BY JULIA STOTZ

SIMON ELEMENT

NEW YORK AMSTERDAM/ANTWERP LONDON TORONTO SYDNEY NEW DELHI

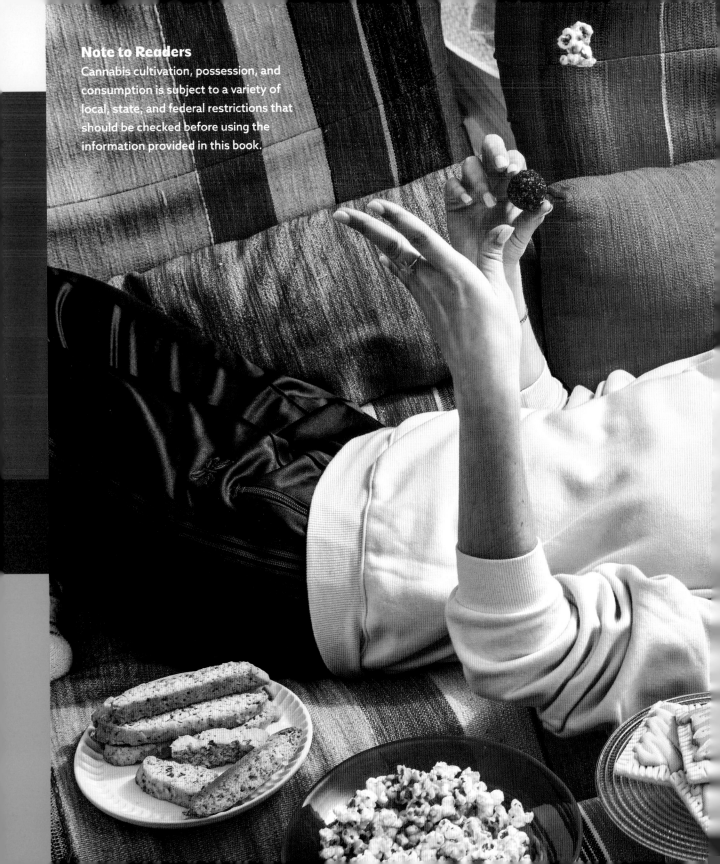

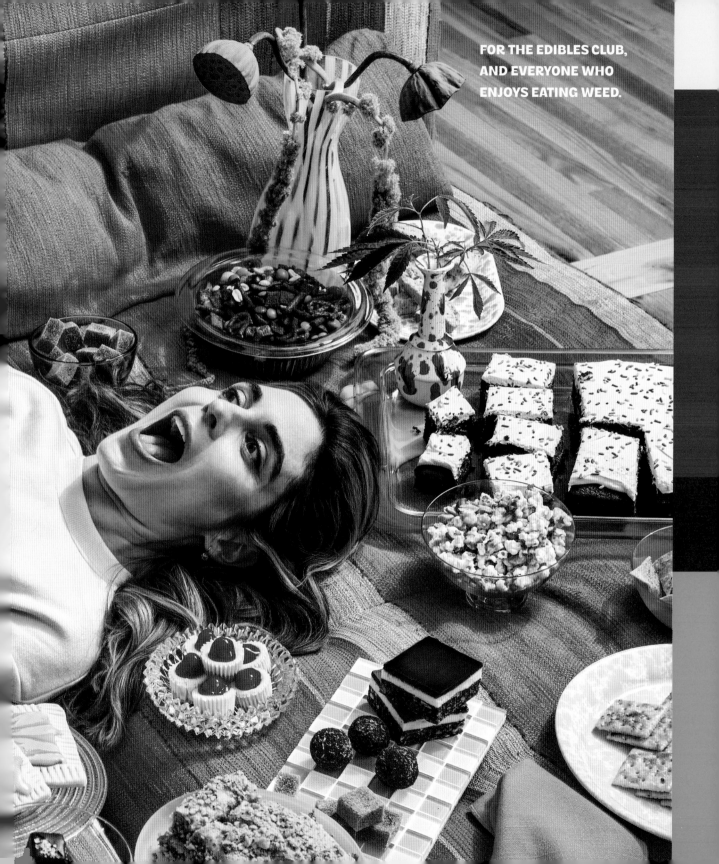

FOR THE EDIBLES CLUB,
AND EVERYONE WHO
ENJOYS EATING WEED.

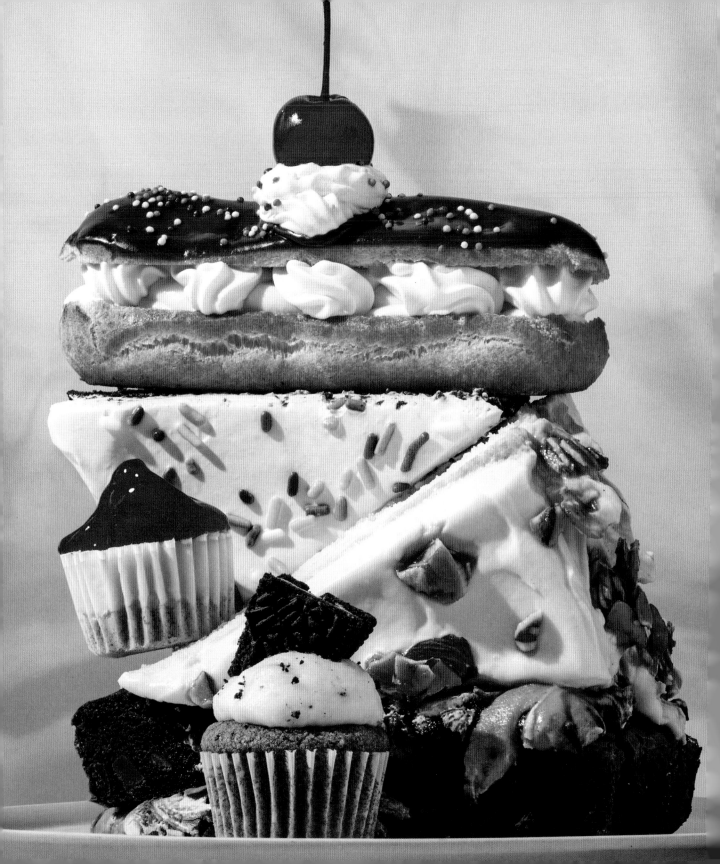

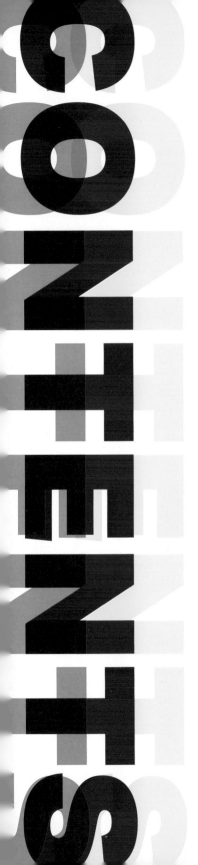

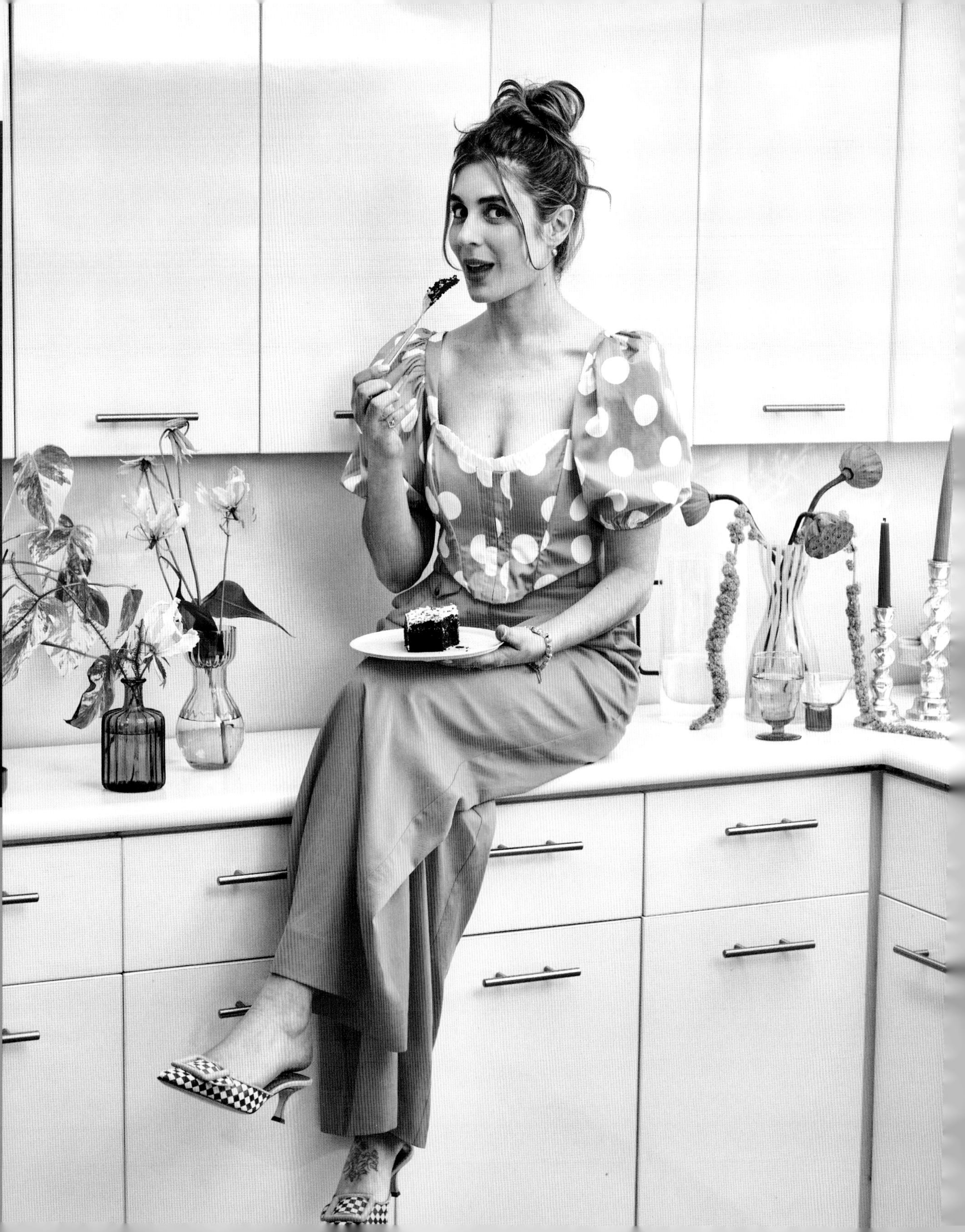

INTRODUCTION

Consider this the definitive guide to cooking with cannabis. With science-backed, stoner-approved recipes, this book will teach you how to infuse edibles quickly and with minimal effort. In the Wild West of pre-legal pot, I mowed through munchies, baked myself out of my mind on pot apple pie, and tossed my cookies in a celebrity's yard. Eventually, I learned how to eat weed responsibly, but it took a lot of work. As weed has become increasingly more accessible, information about how to cook with it has barely budged.

In an industry where professional edible makers have been loath to give up trade secrets and amateurs have been unable to replicate their results, edibles have earned a reputation as unreliable. The science in this book offers, for the first time, lab-tested techniques and shortcuts for using one of the world's most expensive herbs.

I started out as a pothead before earning my cooking chops in Rome. I believe in passing the bowl to everyone, whether it's a handblown glass pipe packed with Durban Poison or vintage Fiestaware filled with my Ganja Guacamole (page 113).

I smoked and ate a lot of pot to write this book. I also ran two hundred lab tests to find the easiest, best, and fastest ways to cook with cannabis. I combined the hard science from those tests, my culinary training, and my decades of experience as a stoner to write *How to Eat Weed & Have a Good Time*. And, like many in my community, my journey to weed began with a Coke can.

LOVE AT FIRST HIT

I spent more of high school flipping upside down for keg stands in Santa Clara frat basements than smoking bowls. At seventeen, with a perpetual spray-tan, pencil-thin eyebrows, and hip-hugging True Religion jeans, I somehow always landed in trouble with drinking. Then, a better option came along.

The previous summer, my cousin and I stole a nug from a house party and hid it in the padding pocket of my push-up bra. We smoked it later, out of a dented Coke can in my grandpa's camper. The high came more from the can fumes than the stale bud. Weed rarely gets first-timers stoned, I learned, eventually.

My friend Michelle knew I was a noob, but she also knew I would do anything to escape another night of watching *Jeopardy!* with my grandma. A lifted Chevy Tahoe pulled up to my house bumping "Ayo for Yayo." As I walked to the car, the passenger's-side window opened, and a thick cloud of skunk-scented white smoke escaped into the night sky. When it cleared, Michelle stuck her head out, grinning like a Cheshire cat, while her chronically red-eyed boyfriend, Craig, puffed deeply on a pipe in the driver's seat. "You gotta smoke some of this, it's hella strong!" Michelle yelled, waving the weed Craig just got with his medical card. "They call it *Romulan*."

I hopped into the back seat, buckled up, and motioned for Craig to drive. My friend took a hit off the pipe and passed it to me. "It's cherry."

Oh shit, I thought to myself. *What the fuck is cherry?* I grew up in a devoutly Christian family; my mom taught religion at my Jesuit high school. When Michelle handed me the pipe, I had no clue what to do.

In the back of Craig's candy-wrapper-strewn SUV, I took a pull and blew out, but made no smoke. "Keep your finger on the carb, dummy," Michelle said, rolling her heavily lined eyes and tugging at the frayed edges of the hole in her jeans. I cringed at myself, put my thumb over the hole on the side of the pipe, took a huge hit, and watched the bowl glow red like a Bing. I held the hot smoke in my chest for a beat, then exhaled and coughed. Time slowed down. My head got light. My body felt like mush. As the car banked on a curvy road, I had an existential moment: When was the last time I said something? How long does this last? Will I ever feel normal again?

Like so many novices before me, I freaked out. My friend intuited my state of mind and suggested we stop at twenty-four-hour Bay Area munchie destination Donut Wheel. As I pushed open the door to the fluorescent-lit bakery, the sugar-soaked air snapped me out of paranoia and hunger kicked in. One bite of an extraordinary maple Long John hooked me. Food sparked my love for weed.

OVERBAKED: MY UNDERWHELMING INTRODUCTION TO EDIBLES

Two years and countless bowls later, my newfound passion for weed fused with my lifelong knack for cooking and I baked my first edible. I knew weed in food existed because my mom told me about the time she ate too many pot brownies while visiting my uncle Ned on Kauai. He left a plate of irresistibly fudgy chocolate bombs on the table without telling her about the special ingredient. My mom's sweet tooth knows no bounds, so she gobbled the entire batch of brownies, one by one.

She told the story as a cautionary tale, followed by a strong warning: Stay away from edibles. I completely disregarded that advice when a greasy-haired UC Santa Cruz dropout handed me a jar of chartreuse fat labeled *XXX*. I grabbed the jar, looked him in his half-drooped eyes, and asked how much cannabutter to use in a pie. He took a giant bong rip, shrugged, and said, "All of it?" Seemed legit.

I whipped up a weed apple pie, incorporating every last glob in the crust. I scarfed two slices before I felt the first wave of an edible high. Even though I had already smoked enough that day to go to Mars, I couldn't resist the herbaceousness of the weed butter and the gooey caramelized apples. Or, maybe, I had the munchies. The apple pot pie crept up on me, peaked midway through the movie, and continued to hit me for the next two days. Though I smoked a lot, nobody told me edibles take an hour to feel, have a way more potent effect, and last substantially longer than smoke. Other than my mom, of course.

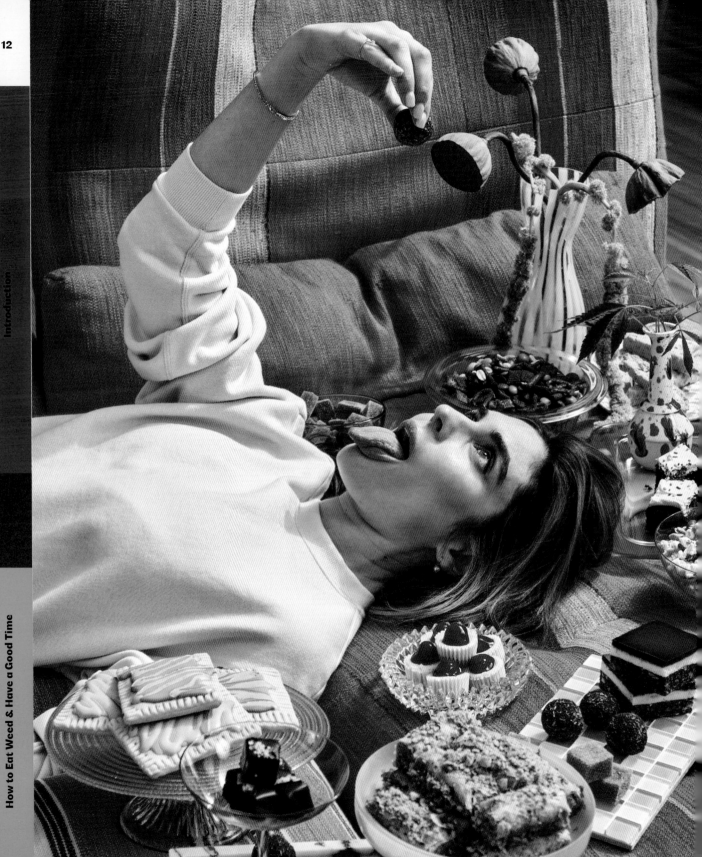

MARY, PATRONESS OF POT

After my apple pie experience, I avoided edibles until I moved to Berkeley and got my first medical card. California's first foray into legal cannabis, Proposition 215, allowed people with a doctor's recommendation to purchase weed and edibles from medical dispensaries. Patients bought weed products by "reimbursing" fellow patients for their time growing and cooking (a legal loophole I would later jump through as an edible maker). In my early twenties, my doctor recommended weed for an eating disorder, a result of anxiety and a lifetime of exposure to WeightWatchers proselytizing. Weed helped—and still helps—me eat more.

Back then, dispensaries carried a handful of edibles, with no standardized dosing system or lab testing. The plastic-wrapped, green-tinged snickerdoodles, skull and crossbones–labeled brownies, and dare-to-nibble gummy bears sold at pot shops guaranteed one thing: couch lock. After one too many sessions of staring at the wall for hours, I saw a hole in the market that I wanted to fill.

Over the years, stoners told me about using trim, aka the small pieces of leaves that get cut off from cannabis flowers after harvest, for cannabutter. Or they'd add it to vodka and stick it in the freezer for months to make a tincture. In 2009, internet resources on edibles instructed similar methods of long infusions, with little to no science backing them up. Some said to pre-toast buds, then infuse them into a fat. Others recommended grinding the buds first, or to add water. Some sternly said not to add water. Whatever the method, they all agreed cooks should definitely plan to spend an entire day working on the infusion. The resulting butter always tasted bitter and green, like oversteeped tea.

Then I met Mary, a statuesque queen-pin from Humboldt with decades of experience growing weed—and cooking it, too.

While working toward my double major at Berkeley, I held jobs as a receptionist at a Victorian bed-and-breakfast, a caretaker for an English professor emeritus, and a salesperson at an upscale, artsy clothing store in Hayes Valley. The boutique's manager, a chic and edgy sales shark by day, became Chloe, a Givenchy-clad, high-end sex worker by night. We often walked to his apartment to smoke together after work, and I would borrow his shoes because we wore the same size. Chloe knew people. When I explained my idea to make fancy edibles, he arranged a trip to visit his grower friend, Mary, at her biodynamic farm a few hours north of the city.

We cruised up the 101, crossing the Golden Gate Bridge and winding through the Valley of the Giants until we reached the Eel River. In the rainy season, the river washed out the piecemeal bridge, so we parked my gold Prius, hopped into a speedboat, and met Mary on the opposite bank. Her wolf dog, Ruby, greeted us with a cold, wet lick as we piled into the back of her truck. I rolled the window down as we drove up to Mary's stilted A-frame and a blast of weed filled the truck, wafting from the Blue Dream and White Widow bushes covering the property. I had arrived at the source, where weed grew as tall as apple trees and branches laden with resinous buds clustered into colas the size of baseball bats.

Mary hosted us for two days. We smoked joint after joint, discussing how to make edibles, the intricacies of astrology, and the perils of working in the weed industry. After decades growing and selling weed, she knew the seedy underbelly of the male-dominated business.

Before we dipped out of California's Green Triangle, Mary handed me a pound of pungent, crystally Blue Dream cold-water hash—what would become my catalyst into the herbaceous world of edibles—and said, "Remember, it ain't over 'til the Clover": a warning to drive by the book until I got to Cloverdale, in Sonoma, where the highway patrol dropped off.

A POT OF MARIGOLD

After my visit to Mary's garden, I experimented with the potent hash, selling micro-dosed confections under the name Marigold Sweets. My discreet packaging and the consistent high struck a chord with wealthy and eccentric Bay Area customers. My clients picked them up while they shopped for Comme des Garçons at the clothing store where I worked. I kept the busted microwave in the bathroom stocked with little black boxes, which I wrapped in dark blue labels printed at FedEx. Inside, hand-folded Florentine paper origami cradled four hash-infused salted caramels, each enrobed in dark chocolate and sprinkled with Maldon sea salt. Shoppers took their stash and left cash in the microwave.

I moved to LA in 2012 and upgraded from sneaking around broken appliances to handing out chocolates to the waitstaff at a legendary hotel on the Sunset Strip as I dined on the patio and rubbed elbows with Katy Perry. While I worked part-time retail jobs and wrote roundups for food websites, word got around Hollywood about the chocolates. The money helped pay for groceries and shoes. After a year, I earned enough for a four-month culinary internship in Rome. While I shaped gnocchi above the Tiber River, Chloe moved the hundreds of boxes I'd packaged before I left.

A few months after I got back to LA, the extremely high boyfriend of a friend recommended I get in touch with a cannabis dispensary called Cornerstone. When I contacted the exclusive medical-use shop and said I'd heard about them through Alex, the owner misunderstood and thought I meant a manager by the same name. In classic stoner form, the bumble led me to a break, and I entered the arena of regulated weed.

Through years of making chocolates for the loyal patients of Cornerstone, I cultivated a deeper knowledge of weed science, cooking with concentrates, and doling out precise doses through lab testing. Previously, I had shied away from publicly promoting my weed—I hadn't even told my family the true nature of my candy business. Now my chocolates lined the shelves of a legit licensed dispensary, and a feature in the *LA Times* helped spread the word.

LES BONG TEMPS

Around the same time, my friend Jessica Koslow (the owner of popular Los Angeles restaurant Sqirl) told a *Vice* producer about my chocolates, recommending me for a weed cooking show called *Bong Appétit.*

I started as a food stylist, but the minute I walked on set with my iron lungs, pixie haircut, and edible know-how, the producers had another idea. They mic'd me up and threw me on camera. I shook off my initial stage fright by connecting to chefs over the flavor profiles of weed. In the first episode, a culinary lightbulb went off when Wes Avila of Guerilla Tacos and I tasted shiso flavors in a weed leaf. I saw the potential to innovate in both the weed and food worlds.

Through three seasons and a James Beard Foundation Award nomination, I infused dishes with cannabis alongside top chefs: I cooked a kush Korean feast with Deuki Hong, served a stoner shabbat with the legendary Joan Nathan, and fried kief loukoumades with Iron Chef Cat Cora for Xzibit. We pimped his dessert with THC. As the show evolved, I stepped up to the plate as a judge alongside host and Cypress Hill leadman B-Real and cannabis chef Miguel Trinidad. The competition format introduced me to chefs from around the world, and I got to smoke with industry legends, taking bong rips with Wiz Khalifa and hitting a multi-joint pipe with George Clinton of the Funkadelic.

Since then, I've created an online cannabis cooking club where I share my stand-and-stir recipe videos with my hungry audience while documenting the burgeoning global edibles scene. Along the way, I tested and learned new techniques for cooking with weed.

I developed recipes that keep dab bros happy at game night and figured out the secret to salves for soothing Grandma's arthritic hands. I whipped up batches of microdosed weed hummus for camping trips, and always remembered to pack the black pepper crackers—just in case someone went ham on the dip (see page 135).

In my decade-plus of medicating and educating people about edibles, I have learned—smoked pot, forgotten, and learned again—everything anyone needs to know about how to eat weed and have a good time.

And, finally, I wrote it all down.

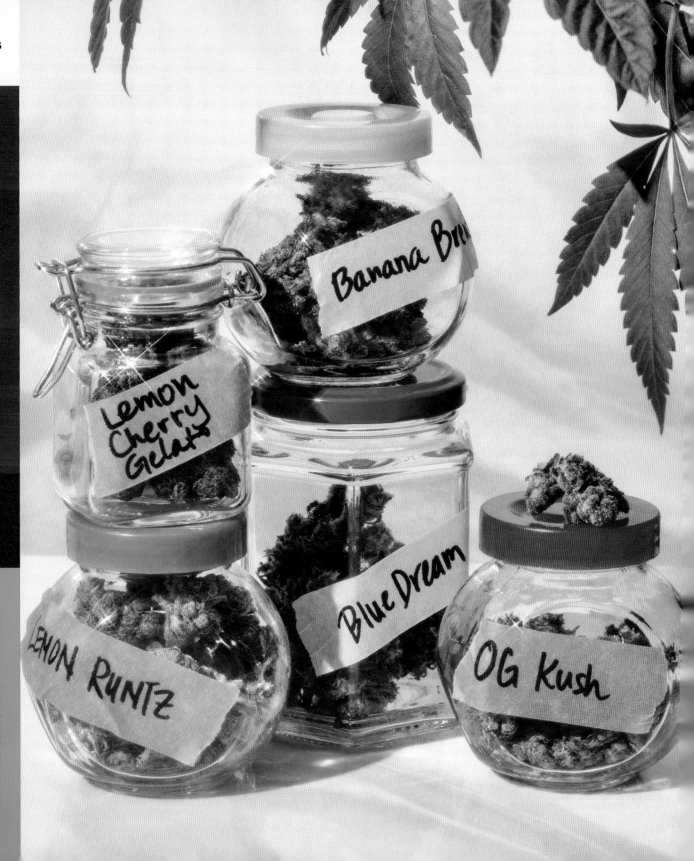

WHAT IS WEED?

Pot, herb, ganja, cannabis: Whatever the name, weed has packed bowls and fueled space cakes for generations. Bill Clinton didn't inhale, Barack Obama did, and Nixon declared a war on it. This potent plant polarized the world into stoners and narcs. Depending on whom you ask and when, the drug fries brains, deepens sleep, or soothes pain. All this magic and power comes from an herb: weed.

THE CHRONIC-LES

Humans have carefully cultivated, toked, and eaten weed for millennia. Native to Central Asia, weed popped up in recorded history as early as 2800 BCE, when Emperor Shennong, the father of Chinese medicine, touted its medicinal uses in his pharmacopeia. He credited the plant with helping to treat gout, rheumatism, malaria, and even absent-mindedness. (And people say stoners are forgetful!) That said, cannabis seeds followed human migration for around twelve thousand years, according to Dr. Marc-Antoine Crocq.

Since the emperor's medicinal discoveries, weed has spread around the globe like mint without a pot. In the 1800s, Irish physician William Brooke O'Shaughnessy introduced it to the Western world and found its potential for aiding children with epilepsy. Humans continue to grow and consume more weed than ever, despite the "Reefer Madness" stoked in the 1930s and perpetuated by the Controlled Substance Act of 1970 labeling it a Schedule One drug—on the same level as heroin.

Eating weed dates as far back as the plant's cultivation and inhalation. In India, Hindus have long celebrated Holi by throwing vibrant colors on one another and drinking bhang lassi, a fruity infused yogurt drink, or bhang thandai, a dosed and saffron-spiced nut milk. The earliest evidence of edibles originates from Morocco, where, after dinner, nomadic tribes served majoun, a spice-laden, hash-laced date-and-nut ball. Alice B. Toklas snuck an adaptation of majoun called "Haschich Fudge" into her eponymous 1954 cookbook and recommended the heady sweet treat as a way to ward off the common cold and for the Ladies' Bridge Club to weed out the turkeys. In the 1980s, Mary Jane Rathbun earned her nickname, Brownie Mary, for baking and donating thousands of magical brownies for AIDS patients in San Francisco at the height of the pandemic.

Today, edibles bake up a big business. From fancy pot-laced chocolates like mine to gummies shaped like Mike Tyson's ear, they come in all flavors, sizes, and doses. As legal weed expands, so too does the demand for edibles—and the hunger for knowledge about how to make them at home.

POT BOTANY

Before we jump into the kitchen, let's learn about our star ingredient.

Weed grows like spinach or kiwi vines: Cannabis generally needs both a male and a female plant to reproduce. It can also "herm out" under stressful conditions, spontaneously turning into a hermaphrodite to reproduce asexually, but the important information for cannabis cooks comes from understanding the plant's sexual reproduction.

The female plant holds all the power. Growers mostly pluck the male plants from the garden as soon as their balls drop, though they'll hold on to the healthiest to cultivate new cannabis strains. By isolating female plants (pistillates) from male plants (staminates), growers prevent pollination. The females use the energy that would have been spent developing seeds to grow bigger flowers.

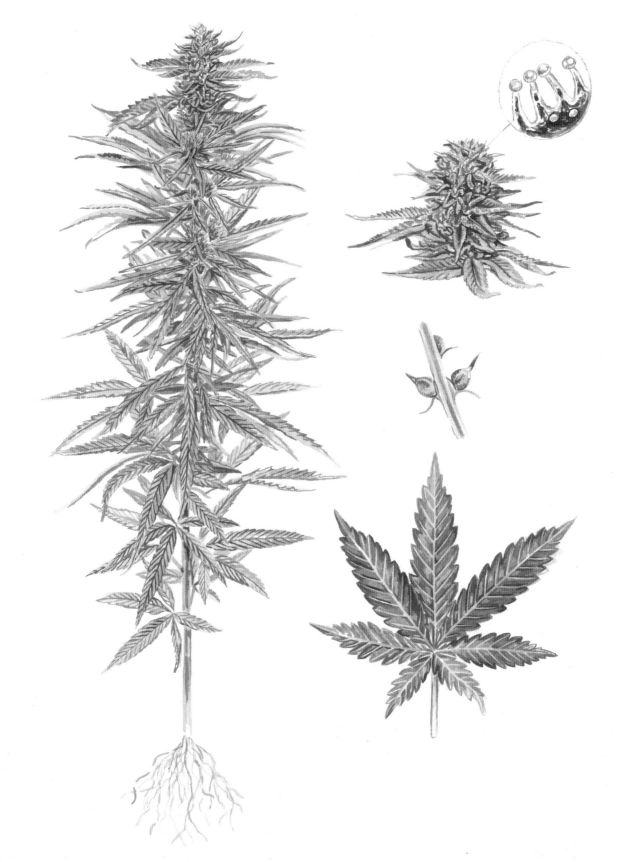

These superpowered female plants are prized for their pungent, trichome-covered flowers. Trichomes, small glandular hairs that concentrate on cannabis flowers, secrete bitter, pungent, and sticky compounds to disorient predators and deter them from eating the plant's reproductive system. The resin they produce also holds the high for humans. The selection and cultivation of plants that grow trichome-laden (sticky-icky) flowers has produced cannabis plants twice as potent as when Cheech and Chong first hit the bong.

Trichomes consist of stalks and gland heads; they usually look like a stick with a balloon on the end. The trichome head fills with cannabis resin, a sap-like substance that contains more than 125 phytocannabinoids, the compounds that give weed its potency, including the potentially psychoactive one: THCA.

When we smoke a joint or hit a bong, the cannabinoids and other compounds vaporize from the heat and activate, entering our lungs to get us high. In order to get high from eating weed, though, we have to heat it through other methods. This is why we activate THCA through a process called decarboxylation, which I'll teach you how to do in the oven or microwave or using sous vide (pages 29–31).

HOW DOES WEED GET US HIGH?

Laughter to the point of peeing, eating multiple sleeves of cookies in a row, forgetting to set the timer for the pot roast: Every stoner knows, generally, what to expect when they get high. Inhale, exhale, cough, and repeat, until it feels like someone hit the slow-motion button. But, from giggle fits to the munchies, weed affects everyone differently, and highs can change between sessions, depending on the strain and the method of consumption.

The more we know about how weed gets us high, the more we can control our well-being and state of mind, setting ourselves up for a fun time getting stoned.

We have one scientist to thank for our knowledge of the active compounds in weed: the grandfather of cannabinoids, Dr. Raphael Mechoulam, who set out to study weed because nobody else could. He saw the huge gaps in research on cannabis, due to its status as a controlled substance, and reached out to his government in Israel for permission to work with it. Not only did the country agree to allow the work but the police also gave him confiscated hash to use for his experiments. His groundbreaking research pinpointed the exact compound that gets us stoned: delta 9-tetrahydrocannabinol, or THC, the compound found to provide the psychoactive effects of weed. His lab went on to discover cannabidiol or CBD, valued for its medicinal benefits. But it would take another twenty years to discover how these plant compounds worked in our bodies.

Later labs identified the receptors found all over the body that control the effects of cannabis. This collection of receptors for cannabinoids is called the endocannabinoid system (ECS). While stoners would like to believe we have an ECS because we need weed, we actually naturally produce our own endocannabinoids—including the delight-fully named "bliss molecule," or anandamide. When we use cannabis, its phytocannabinoids also fit into the little ECS receptors that run all over our body, even down to our bones.

The ECS regulates a majority of our bodily functions, including appetite. It's the reason that after you hit a bong, you hit In-N-Out. Once THC enters our lungs and travels to our brain, it sets off the CB1 receptors, which stimulates the release of ghrelin, the "hunger hormone," according to the *Journal of Biological Chemistry*. The ECS also controls anxiety (hello, paranoia!) and sleep, the latter of which is the top reason people tell me they love edibles. Laws have so far inhibited research into how cannabis interacts with our bodies. With the changing legal landscape, though, there's hope more good science will follow.

DO STRAINS EVEN MATTER?

Blue Dream, Durban Poison, White Widow, and OG Kush: Like apples, hops, or grapes, weed comes in many cultivars, usually described as strains. Traditionally, potheads divide strains into two categories: indica and sativa. Indica plants grow shorter, faster, with more buds, while sativa plants grow taller with longer fan leaves. Stoner wisdom says to seek out sativa strains for a more upbeat, zippy high, and *indica* means "in-da-couch." But, at this point, pure sativa or indica hardly exist: Most strains blend into a sativa-dominant or indica-dominant cultivar. Seed collectors hunt for pure strains and locally adapted seeds from around the world, cultivated for generations by growers dedicated to preserving genetics, such as cannabis activist Aram "Kodam" Limsakul.

On an island in the Gulf of Thailand called Koh Tao, he follows in the footsteps of his mother, grandmother, and previous generations, cultivating cannabis, including a mango sativa you can smell from a foot away. Myrcene, the terpene responsible for the fruity aroma, packs a powerful sedative effect. Ko Dam rolled me a joint and we puffed on the sweet buds while walking through his tropical garden speckled with avocado trees and other psychotropic plants. The high from his pure sativa flower felt euphoric.

Terpenes are the building blocks of essential oils. They are what make them smell. Their aromas attract pollinators and, in the case of cannabis, repel predators. They spritz out of the zested rinds of lemons and define the scent of rosemary. Some even alter the color, as in anthocyanin, the water-soluble flavonoid responsible for purple cauliflower, red berries, and violet weed like Purple Kush. Like heirloom roses, each cannabis strain produces a unique aroma from its combination of terpenes and flavonoids.

Weed with pungent terpenes or flavonoids, from high-quality growing conditions and expert curing of flowers to preserve the aroma, is considered "loud," and it's a good thing. When weed loses its loudness, the more volatile terpenes and flavonoids have evaporated. Temperature can be a major factor in this: Some evaporate at temperatures as low as 70ºF and most start to degrade at 100ºF. Storing weed flowers in a cool dark place in an airtight jar helps to maintain the volatile and precious terpenes.

On *Bong Appétit*, we had a pantry filled with jars of weed, which the chefs smelled to select the strains that worked best with their menu. Using Chocolope, a rich, coffee-flavored flower, enhanced the infused brownies I whipped up for the slumber party episode. Be creative!

Strains of weed, like grape varieties in wine, are a complex puzzle. Cannabis contains a complicated molecular profile, producing more than a hundred phytocannabinoids and a vast array of terpenes and flavonoids in each strain. *The entourage effect* sounds like a reference to the early aughts, but the term actually describes how THC's posse of terpenes, flavonoids, and other phytocannabinoids interact with one another and, together, with our endocannabinoid system. To put it simply, the total effect is not the same as the sum of its parts.

When we smoke, the trip from our lungs through the blood-brain barrier is more direct than when we eat weed. Depending on how we consume it, the terpenes in a cannabis strain might impact the high. When we eat a particular strain, its terpenes hit a number of biological checkpoints where they may get filtered out. Which means that in the kitchen, I use terpenes as more of an additional flavor component than a way to orchestrate the high.

TERPENES

TERPENES	BOILING POINTS	IN FOOD	AROMA	IN STRAINS
LINALOOL	388°F (198°C)	LAVENDER, BAY LAUREL, BASIL	FLORAL	AMNESIA HAZE + LAVENDER KUSH
MYRCENE	334°F (168°C)	MANGO, LEMONGRASS, HOPS	MUSKY + EARTHY	OG KUSH + DURBAN POISON
LIMONENE	349°F (176°C)	ORANGE, LEMONS, CARAWAY	CITRUS + ZESTY	SOUR DIESEL + DO-SI-DOS
PINENE	311°F (155°C)	ROSEMARY, DILL, PARSLEY, BASIL	PINE + FOREST	BLUE DREAM + JACK HERER
CARYOPHYLLENE	320°F (160°C)	PEPPER, CLOVES, SAGE, OREGANO	SPICY + PEPPERY	GELATO + GIRL SCOUT COOKIES
HUMULENE	388°F (198°C)	HOPS, CORIANDER, GINGER	WOODY + EARTHY	WHITE WIDOW + HEADBAND

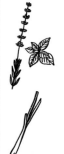

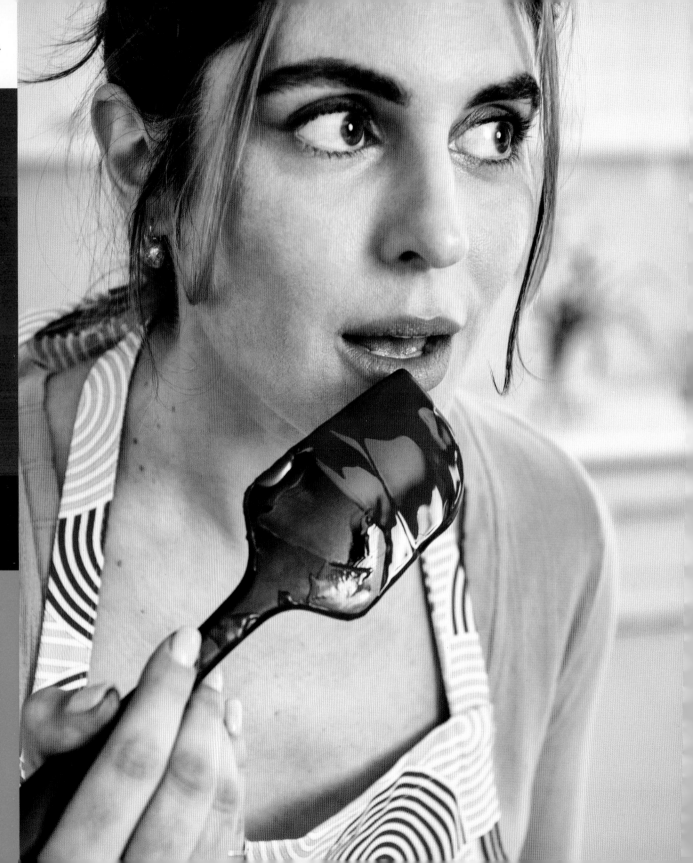

HOW TO
EAT WEED

Weed can make food taste better—plus, nobody ever complains about the smell of brownies. Edibles last longer and feel stronger than smoking, and they require less weed. They minimize pain, deepen sleep, and, when properly dosed, maintain that high, like an extended-release version of THC.

Don't get me wrong: I love smoking weed, but edibles, while not always healthful, keep our lungs out of the equation. When I first started selling chocolates, I quickly learned that much of the audience for my treats rarely smoked or couldn't smoke. Edibles offer a tastier and more healthful high for everyone.

BONGS VERSUS BROWNIES

At first, people often approach edibles with excitement: The idea of eating something and getting high at the same time feels like two birds, everyone stoned. Except the anticipation makes people impatient, and they question the efficacy of such a disarmingly delicious treat. So, they take another bite, just in case the weed didn't work. By the time the first nibble hits, sometimes several hours later, they've polished off the entire cookie.

When the tiny delta-9-THC (Δ^9-THC) molecule enters our lungs in a puff of pot smoke, it makes a beeline for our bloodstream and quickly slips through the blood-brain barrier. The semipermeable membrane shields us from toxic substances, and, fortunately, cannabinoids don't count as such. So, when we smoke, the high hits us almost instantaneously and allows us to control or titrate the effects easily. Not high enough? Smoke more. Too high? Stop smoking.

With edibles, the Δ^9-THC takes a longer trip. First, while we chew, some cannabinoids reach the bloodstream through the mucous membranes under the tongue. The rest travel down to the stomach and through the liver, which weeds out any harmful substances before they release into the entire bloodstream. It uses enzymes to metabolize the Δ^9-THC into 11-hydroxy-THC, a molecule even more adept at binding to CB1 receptors than Δ^9-THC. All this digesting takes far longer than inhaling, so edibles take longer to kick in than smoked cannabis. But the conversion to 11-hydroxy-THC also makes edibles feel stronger and last longer.

I once gave an overworked friend a box of chocolates with a very stern warning to start with only half of a chocolate, then wait at least an hour to feel the effects. I explained, in the clearest terms possible, that, should he still not feel anything, he needed to wait another hour before eating the other half. He waited fifteen minutes before polishing off the entire box. The next day, his housekeeper found him passed out, the candy wrappers scattered all over the floor.

When I asked him why he didn't listen, he said that the chocolate tasted too good and had zero pot flavor, so when the high took too long to kick in, he doubted my skills. The lesson here is to never doubt my skills. And, also, to wait at least an hour for an edible to kick in.

ACTIVATE THE HIGH

At a weed-infused Super Bowl party in one of West Hollywood's many McMansions, a six-foot-tall, leather-clad biker bro picked up a nug of Sour Diesel, scooped it through the infused spinach dip, and shoved it into his mouth. The group of weed influencers around him widened their bloodshot eyes in shock, thinking the whole nug would get him more blazed than a wildfire on a windy day. But eating that raw weed likely got him more constipated than high: Fresh weed needs to be heated to activate the buzz.

With smoked cannabis, the heat comes from the hot cherry slowly burning down the end of a joint or on top of a bowl. Heat detaches a carboxyl group from the raw acidic cannabinoids, most notoriously THCA and CBDA, in a process called decarboxylation. That releases carbon dioxide (CO_2) and transforms the cannabinoids into their more stable—and psychoactive—forms: THC and CBD.

THC becomes psychotropic, while CBD becomes anxiolytic and anti-inflammatory.

Decarboxylation occurs commonly in the world: in the fermentation of wine, when cheese ripens, and even with each breath we take. Whenever carbon dioxide gets released, that is decarboxylation.

Old-school edibles, like the ones my aunty Yo on Kauai makes, call for throwing raw shake directly into a recipe, like classic brownie batter. The weed decarboxylates while the brownies bake, but only partially—around 30 to 40 percent, depending on the recipe. The crunchy grass can get stuck in your teeth, too, but it gets the job done in a pinch.

Other techniques combine decarboxylation with infusion, like slow-cooker coconut oil, which takes several hours longer than the two processes done separately. The long infusion time also extracts more of the bitter green chlo-

THCA

TETRAHYDROCANNABINOLIC ACID

DECARBOXYLATION
RELEASE OF CO_2

THC

DELTA-9-TETRAHYDROCANNABINOL

rophyll flavor and other acrid compounds found in the plant.

In a shocking turn of events, the internet contains a lot of wrong information about how to decarboxylate weed. A plethora of online how-to videos and recipes show people throwing weed onto a sheet pan, covering it with foil (or not), and baking it until the nugs turn from verdant green to crispy brown.

While browned food usually tastes best, the blasts of heat from the oven dry out the buds and destroy the terpenes—those volatile essential oils found in fruit, vegetables, and herbs, such as weed (see page 21). Whereas a little char enhances oven-roasted broccoli, overly crispy weed turns bitter and can actually degrade the THC into CBN, a compound that contributes to the soporific nature of weed. The oxygen binds to the hydrogen molecules in THC to make H_2O and leaves behind CBN. To make extra-sleepy edibles, I intentionally degrade weed by heating it for a longer time and exposing the buds to air.

To avoid nappy-time weed, remove oxygen from the equation. In the oven or microwave, do this by wrapping the weed in parchment paper, which prevents the resin in the weed from sticking to the silicon or foil. Put in a heat-safe reusable silicone bag (or foil, if in the oven) and try to knock out all the air from the bag before heating. Alternatively, sous vide cooking decarboxylates the pot without any degradation.

What if...?

For decarboxylating larger amounts of pot (¼ ounce or more), increase the time by 20 percent for each process and burp the bag (release the built-up gas) halfway through.

The freshness of the weed will also impact the time needed to fully decarboxylate the flower. If the weed feels very fresh and sticky, as if it has more moisture, add extra time. If the flower is more than six months old or feels crumbly and dry, decarb for less time.

For information about decarboxylation of concentrates, see page 37.

Oven Decarboxylation

One of the simplest methods for decarboxylation uses the oven. For spotty ovens, use an oven thermometer to monitor the temperature.

1   /   Preheat the oven to 245°F.

2   /   Create a parchment paper pouch around the weed or hash and slip it into a heat-safe silicone bag or foil pouch.

3   /   To protect the flower from blasts of heat and limit oxygen exposure, smash out as much air as possible from the silicon pouch or foil, then seal it. If using foil, fold tightly.

4   /   Bake for 40 minutes; after 30 minutes, more than 90 percent of THCA activates into stoney THC.

Convection Oven Decarboxylation

To speed up the process, use a convection oven. Follow the same steps as above, but decrease the temperature to 220ºF and bake for just 20 minutes.

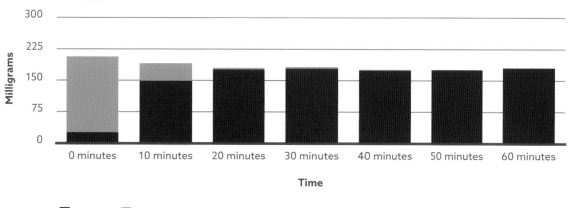

Oven Decarboxylation Rate 245°F

Milligrams — Time

■ THC   ▨ THCA

Sous Vide Decarboxylation

The gentlest way to activate the high of cannabis enlists a culinary nerd's favorite appliance: an immersion circulator, aka a sous vide device. It best protects the terpenes and ensures the weed won't degrade during decarboxylation, though it requires more setup with the vacuum sealer, more work with the burping, and a longer decarboxylation time. The controlled water bath decarboxylates the weed, and the vacuum seal completely prevents degradation. As the graph below illustrates, after 45 minutes, nearly 90 percent of the THC activates, though it takes more than 2 hours for full conversion.

When using this method for larger amounts of weed, gas released in the bag can cause the bag to rise to the surface of the water. Using a resealable sous vide bag allows you to release the gas by "burping" the bag halfway through the process, avoiding this issue.

1 / Set up an immersion circulator in a water bath and bring the temperature to 200°F.

2 / Create a parchment paper pouch around the weed or hash and slip it into a resealable sous vide bag.

3 / Add pie weights or other heavy items to the bag and vacuum seal it.

4 / Submerge in the water bath for 45 minutes, then open the bag, release the trapped gases, and reseal it. Place it back in the water bath for 45 more minutes.

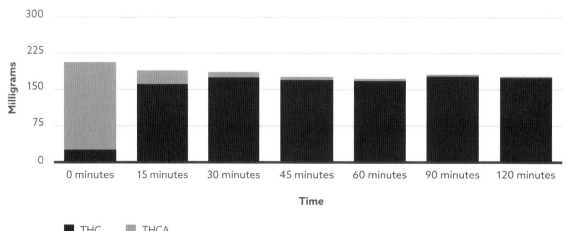

Sous Vide Decarboxylation Rate

Microwave Decarboxylation

The key is to treat heating weed like heating chocolate: short pulses and less time than it takes to open a child-resistant container.

1 / Create a parchment paper pouch around the weed or hash and slip it into a microwave-safe silicone bag.

2 / Roll the bag up, pushing out as much air as possible before sealing.

3 / Check the wattage of your microwave. For wattage lower than 1050 watts, increase the time by 15 to 30 seconds. For higher wattage, decrease the time by 15 to 30 seconds.

4 / Place the silicone bag in the center of the microwave and microwave on high in 10-second pulses for 1 minute 30 seconds total. If the weed is very fresh, add an additional 15 to 30 seconds.

Decarboxylation to Infusion

Now for the time-saving techniques that illustrate how easy it is to cook with weed.

After decarboxylating your weed, the next step involves one of three options, as laid out in the Mother Infusions section (page 56). One option: Infuse into a fat such as butter, oil, or milk. Another option: Extract into alcohol. Or, finally, simply add ground-up herb directly to a recipe. I recommend using only the whole flower in flavorful recipes like my Queso Extra Fundido (page 120) or Sticky Icky Pot-Stickers (page 106), where the greenness of the ganja harmonizes with a symphony of other herbs and spices.

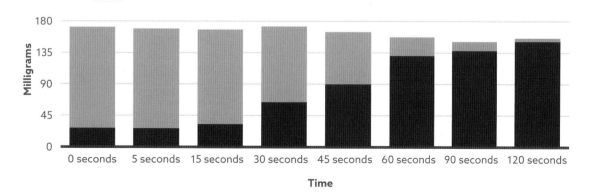

Microwave Decarboxylation Rate
1050 Watts

Milligrams (y-axis): 0, 45, 90, 135, 180

Time (x-axis): 0 seconds, 5 seconds, 15 seconds, 30 seconds, 45 seconds, 60 seconds, 90 seconds, 120 seconds

■ THC   ■ THCA

Special Equipment

A chocolatier needs a dipping fork to hand-enrobe chocolates. A confectioner must have a precise thermometer to monitor the sugar temperature stage. And an edible maker requires a milligram scale to dose correctly. Most kitchen scales struggle to accurately measure ingredients that weigh less than a gram. Since weed weighs very little but contains hundreds of milligrams of potency per gram, home cannabis cooks need more precise scales. Anyone who bought weed from the living room of their dealer knows the small, usually black jewelry scale used to weigh out dime bags and eighths. A jewelry scale works for smaller amounts of flower or concentrates, but a larger high-precision scale allows cooks to weigh a gram of flower and a cup of flour on the same machine. I recommend a Bonvoisin Lab Analytical Balance 500g x .001g High Precision Lab Scale (available online anywhere lab equipment is sold).

To decarboxylate the weed by sous vide, I recommend using a resealable sous vide bag or a resealable silicone bag (such as a Stasher bag) so you can evacuate the carbon dioxide released during decarboxylation. When you are decarbing large amounts of flower or concentrate in a sous vide, CO_2 builds up, and you need to either cut and reseal a standard sous vide bag, use one with a valve to let the gas escape, or use a resealable silicone bag and burp it; otherwise, you risk an explosion.

All the infusions and recipes in this book call for ground decarboxylated flower. Most stoners have a designated weed grinder to avoid cross contamination. A sharp kitchen knife also works well to chop up the weed; just be sure to clean the blade with food-grade alcohol to remove resin.

Legalization has brought to market machines designed to make everything you want to do with weed easier, including infusion and decarboxylation machines. While I have plenty of pastry tools, I don't like single-use machines. It's a personal preference, but I don't have a ton of space in my kitchen, and decarboxylation at home is really easy, like making a pot of coffee—another task with plenty of fun gizmos and gadgets to use.

COOKING WITH CONCENTRATES

Some weed products enable cooks to skip infusion and even decarboxylation through the process of concentrating the plant's resin. Concentrates wield incredible amounts of potential potency. When we invited pizzaiolo Frank Pinello from Best Pizza to throw some pizzas on *Bong Appétit*, everyone loved the idea of adding a concentrate called terp sauce, or "sauce," to the tomato sauce. Sauce isolates the THCA in raw weed along with the terpenes, removes everything else, then blends the cannabinoids and terpenes back together into a potent, aromatic goop. It's basically cannabis essential oil. The show's in-house cannabis expert, Ry Prichard, poured an overly generous glug of sauce into the lightly seasoned puréed tomatoes. Frank baked the margherita pizzas for a packed house of celebrity skateboarders in a very hot oven, igniting the THCA. Everyone gnawed down on infused slices except for me, because I knew what was in store.

My years of cooking with concentrates and decarbing while I cook (see pages 29–31) taught me that the intense heat of the pizza oven would activate a decent amount of the sauce in the pizza, making these hyper-potent pies. By skipping the pizza, I avoided the terp-burps from the sauce and stuck to the cannabutter garlic knots and the homemade ricotta cannoli infused with the legend-

Concentrates

Types	Average Potency	Solvents	Raw/Decarbed	Form
Kief	40% to 70%	Solventless	Raw	Dry Sift
Hash	50% to 80%	Solventless/Water	Raw	Bubble, Finger, Pressed, Temple Balls
Live Rosin	70% to 90%	Solventless	Raw	Badder, Diamonds, Sauce
Full Extract Oil	50% to 70%	Ethanol	Decarbed	Oil
Butane Hash Oil	70% to 90%	Butane	Raw	Sauce, Budder, Badder, Crumble, Shatter, Crystals
Live Resin	70% to 90%	Butane and Propane	Raw	Sauce, Budder, Badder, Crumble, Shatter, Crystals
Distillate	80% to 95%	Butane, Hexane, Propane, Ethanol, or CO_2	Decarbed	Oil
Isolate	90% to 99%	Butane, Hexane, Propane, or Ethanol	Raw or Decarbed	Diamonds, Crystalline, Powder

ary Frenchy Cannoli hash. The next morning, even our seasoned cannabis producer admitted we put too much sauce in the sauce. But, when used carefully, cannabis concentrates easily melt into recipes without infusion or the need to strain out plant matter, and they make dosing a snap.

What Is a Concentrate?

Concentrates are refined forms of cannabis, which, as the name implies, hyper-concentrate the best parts of cannabis into the smallest volumes. They pack a potency of anywhere from 50 percent for kiefs and hashes to upwards of 90 percent for distillates. As a cook, I think of concentrates like sugar. In its plant form, sugarcane contains a lot of fibrous material to chew through. The crushed sugarcane becomes a juice, which is refined into pure granulated sugar. Similarly, weed concentrates use different methods of extraction to remove plant impurities while isolating the cannabinoids and terpenes found in cannabis. Buying granulated sugar at the store saves a ton of work over buying sugarcane and refining it at home: You skip dealing with the plant matter and putting in the elbow grease, and end up with a more usable product.

Legalization sparked the imagination of cannabis chemists, who distilled, winterized, isolated, and whipped, developing new concentrates to smoke or dab. Those concentrates fall into two categories: solventless and solvent-extracted.

Solventless Concentrates

Solventless concentrates use agitation, extreme cold, or pressure to separate plant matter from the precious, potent resin. Old-school finger hash sticks to the digits of trimmers and gets rolled into snakes to twist into a joint or spliff. The dry sift that breaks off when mashing weed through the metal claws of a grinder, falls through the screen, and collects in the lower level is a type of kief. More sophisticated processes sift kief through finer screens, use colder temperatures to produce bubble (or ice-water) hash, and squash out the oil from fresh-frozen flower to make live rosin.

The more skilled a concentrate maker, the less plant matter ends up in the final concentrate. The goal: trichomes only. Hash, for example, is graded on a six-star rating system, filtered through fine micron screens that separate the pure trichome heads and stalks and leave behind the rest of the plant matter. One- and two-star hashes contain more detritus or undesirable plant material that smokes when heated, rather than bubbling and melting. Three- and four-star hash or halfmelt hash tops bowls and coats the outside of joints but rarely gets dabbed, because too much plant material still remains in the concentrate. (Dabbing is inhaling vaporized concentrate.) When burned or dabbed, six-star hash bubbles and fully melts, without leaving behind any residue. Most edible makers use half-melt or lower quality hash, because cooking with full-melt hash would be like using Wagyu steak to make beef jerky.

Solvent-Extracted Concentrates

A solvent is any compound that dissolves a solute into a solution. Technically, cannabutter and tincture are solvent-extracted, because the solvents (butter and alcohol) extract the resin from the

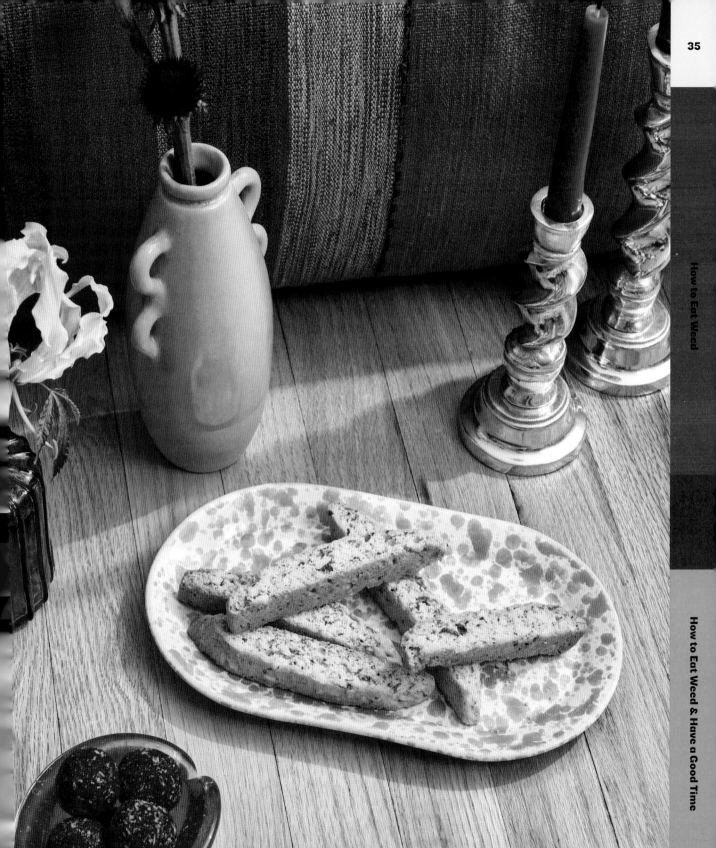

plant. Commercially extracted concentrates use more powerful substances, such as carbon dioxide, ethanol, hexane, butane, or propane, to separate the cannabinoids and terpenes. Live resin, similar to live rosin, starts with fresh-frozen flower, but instead of squishing the oils out, it uses butane to extract the oils. Other concentrates start from cured flower, but either way, the solvents dissolve the resin from the plant, converting it into a crude cannabis oil. Then, through various methods and depending on the end goal, the oil gets further purified, refined, and turned into a range of products.

For some concentrates, that means purification through winterization, which deep-chills the resin until the terpenes and other plant matter divide into layers that are easily separated from the cannabinoids. Distillation heats and vaporizes all the cannabinoids. They capture those now decarboxylated cannabinoids in an oil. Isolates take that one step further, removing everything except the THC: They taste like nothing but feel like pure high.

Terpene-rich concentrates take the solvent-extracted hash oil and heat it to specific temperatures, then use mostly proprietary tricks (such as beating it with a handheld mixer or letting it sit in a solvent for a month) to make waxes, shatter, sauces, budders, badders, diamonds, and sugars. These concentrates take their names from the characteristics created during the extraction process. They are mostly consumed by dabbing, because of their loud flavor profiles. I typically stay away from terpene-heavy, solvent-based concentrates such as live resin or the terp sauce with which Frank made pizza. I find eating large amounts of terpenes similar to eating soap or overly floral candy.

Full-Spectrum Concentrates versus Distilled Concentrates

Concentrates in which all the terpenes, flavonoids, and cannabinoids stay together in the final product are known as full-spectrum. Solventless full-spectrum concentrates, such as hash, kief, live rosin, and full-extract cannabis oil, preserve the unique aromas and flavors of each strain. When cooking with full-spectrum concentrates, dose lightly and try to cook with terpene profiles that will complement the recipe: A Garlic Kush live rosin will taste better in the Oregano Marinara (page 118) than the Silly Vanilly Wafers (page 175).

The opposite of full-spectrum concentrates are clear distillate and pure forms of THCA (or CBDA) isolate. In these, all plant matter, terpenes, and flavonoids are completely removed, leaving only cannabinoids. These concentrates deliver a consistent high with undetectable flavor, making them ideal for precise, even dosing, like in a professional kitchen.

When I make larger batches or need to dose a recipe more potently, I use decarbed concentrates like distillate. Distilling decarboxylates the cannabis, allowing home cooks to skip a step, and simplifies dosing even further. With a decarboxylated concentrate, the only math required is to calculate how much oil to use based on the potency and total desired milligrams in a batch.

With my salted caramels, a small batch makes 64 chocolates. California (and most states with legal cannabis industries) sets the maximum dose at

10 milligrams per serving, with a 10 percent margin for error. That means if I dose each chocolate at 10 milligrams, I can be off by only 1 milligram on each chocolate. If I used shake or trim to make a cannabutter for my caramels, hitting that 10-milligram limit on every batch would require a lot more lab testing. But using .8 of a gram of 80 percent concentrate means that 600 mg of THC spreads evenly among the chocolates and each ends up with 10 milligrams.

Think of cooking with flower as the Luddite version of making edibles: You do everything from scratch, and it is impressive when executed well. But even Ina Garten knows that sometimes store-bought saves enough time and makes little enough difference in the final product to be worthwhile.

Decarboxylation of Concentrates

To decarboxylate raw concentrates such as hash and kief, use the same methods as described here for flower. More viscous concentrates, such as live rosin and live resin, require a lower temperature. Decarboxylate them in an oven-safe glass bowl covered with foil at 220°F for about 1 hour, or until the oil stops bubbling (releasing CO_2).

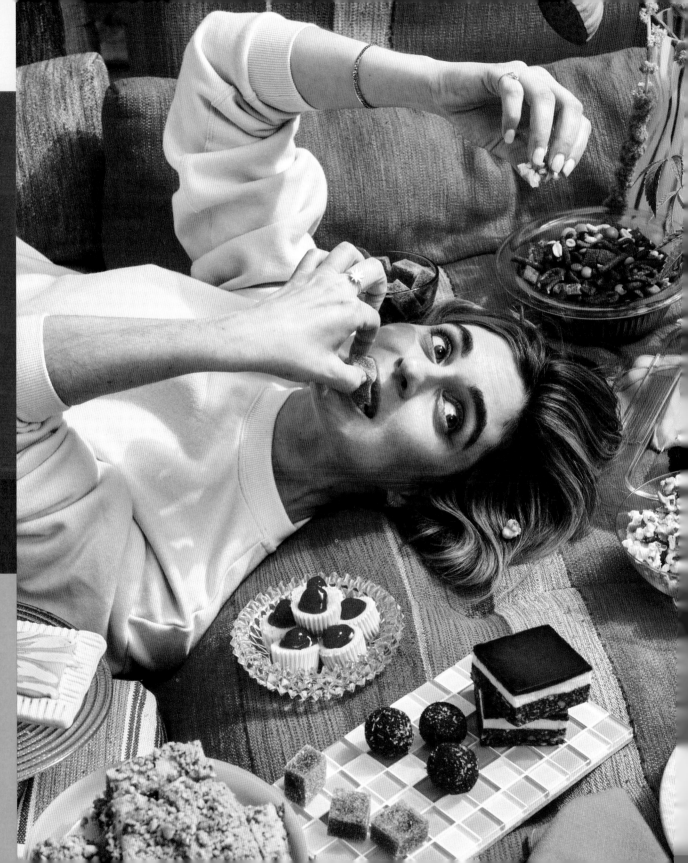

...AND HAVE A GOOD TIME

The second part of this book's title matters just as much (if not more) than the first: Eating weed should go hand in hand with having a good time. This section provides a road map for fun, with tips for buying and storing weed, a formula for an ethical dose, and a few cautionary tales to help you sidestep the oft-repeated mistakes of rookie edible makers.

HOW TO BUY WEED

Most people start off buying weed from a guy in a garage where the nugs come in zip-top bags that were decanted from mason jars stuffed with pot grown in his closet. Meanwhile, at fancy weed shops that have popped up everywhere from LA to Bangkok, budtenders explain their favorite strains, offer a wide array of edibles, and show off a full slate of accurately dosed cannabis commodities.

To purchase a cannabis product at a dispensary in the United States, there are two things you need to bring with you: a valid form of identification and cash, because, at the moment, most shops only take cash. Usually, a security guard will greet you at the door—remember this industry deals with expensive products in large quantities, like a jewelry store, and they have to protect the goods. Expect to pay a significant amount of tax on top of the base price: Every regulation involved in legal pot costs money. Think of it as paying to know you won't smoke moldy greens or eat edibles with contaminants. Weed products go through more rigorous testing than the food in grocery stores.

Shelves are sorted into categories: flower, edibles, pills, sublinguals, concentrates, and topicals. Every shop will have different brands and products, with signs indicating any discounts and specials on the flashy packages. In Canada, they have pot shops in the malls, but, due to regulations there, the products all come in muted packaging.

The best bit of advice I can offer for buying weed is to talk to the people working at the dispensary. The budtenders live, breathe, and smoke this stuff—one of the perks of the job is an unlimited supply of weed and free samples. Ask them for well-priced flower or concentrates to cook with and if they have any strains they're really excited about—much like you might ask a farmer about produce at the farmer's market. A good budtender will listen to your goals and point you in the right direction. If you're looking for a strain high in peppery beta-caryophyllene to infuse the Cannabis Chai (page 151), they might recommend Girl Scout Cookies or Gelato.

Buying Weed for Edibles

The weed I buy for smoking and the weed I buy for baking differ in quality and price. When I smoke, I hunt for the skunkiest, gassiest strains to smack me in the face. I smoke higher quality, dense buds packed with trichomes—the resin glands of weed, which produce the high.

For edibles, I use trim or shake and sniff it in search of strains that complement both savory and sweet recipes, such as fruity Blue Dream or lemony Do-Si-Dos—or, if I have a particular recipe in mind, a strain that brings out the flavors of that dish.

Leafly (www.leafly.com) curates an online database of all known strains of weed, their terpene profiles, and purported strain-specific effects, which helps with researching before going to the pot shop. In the Oregano Marinara (page 118), a strain like Garlic Breath plays on the garlic in the sauce. (Plus, it's fun to say, "I made the marinara with Garlic Breath flower.") Once there, trust the budtender to help you find what you need.

Once I find the flower or concentrate, I look at the potency on the label to figure out how much I'll need to make a recipe. In legal states, lab testing provides an estimate of the cannabinoid potency, but take the numbers on the label with a grain of salt and use caution. Labs take a very small sample from a very large batch, and the range in potency from one bud to the next varies drastically across pounds of flower.

Each label will list the potency as a percentage of THC, which is equal to the number of milligrams per gram of product. So, flower labeled 25 percent THCA contains 250 milligrams of THCA per gram of flower. For a more in-depth explanation of THC and dosing, read through the Easy Dose It section below before shopping.

The potency functions the same way with concentrates, except decarboxylated concentrates (like distillate) will provide a THC percentage. For raw concentrates like live rosin, the percentage will refer to the amount of THCA. If you plan to make edibles from concentrates, review the chart of the different types of concentrates (page 33), average potency, and decarboxylation status. Oils, like full-extract cannabis oil, are usually sold in a pipette, while hashes, sauces, and other concentrates generally come in small glass jars.

Each state has limits on the amount of weed a shopper is allowed to purchase at once. I recommend buying smaller amounts at a time, because weed decarboxylates and degrades over time, even at room temperature, unless you smoke an ounce a week (like, um, me). Even so, I look forward to every trip to the pot shop, where I geek out over recipes and new strains with my fellow stoners.

EASY DOSE IT: LESS IS MORE

At the ripe age of twelve, I raided my grandma's liquor cabinet, mixing crème liqueurs, schnapps, and fruity cordials into one syrupy, purple-brown concoction. I gulped it down and declared myself a mixologist. An hour later, I ralphed.

After many more failed attempts to combine alcohols and drink my age in shots, by the time I was legally allowed to drink, I had learned how to moderate. The same lesson applies to cooking with weed. But when people eat too much weed, they rarely pick up an edible again. People give alcohol another shot because drinking feels fun until it doesn't; feeling too high never feels fun.

A consistent, reliable dose is the guiding principle of cooking with weed. People trust their weed cook to take them on a trip and control the high, but to do that, they need to understand how dosing works.

Patience, Young Grass-Chomper

Most states with legal cannabis limit edibles to 10 milligrams of THC per serving. For first-timers, I recommend starting with 2 to 3 milligrams, tops, and eating them on an empty stomach, followed by a light meal. If they don't feel anything after an hour or two, they should wait until the next day to try again, increasing the dose by 1 milligram each day until they slowly find their dose. This process, called titrating, is difficult with edibles, because of how long they take to kick in.

As any seasoned stoner will confirm, an edible high feels awfully different from smoking a bowl, most notably in its strength, which lasts for several hours rather than a few minutes (see more on page 26). High-tolerance stoners, those few who gobble down 100 milligrams without skipping a beat, should focus on cooking with concentrates (page 33). And, of course, mistakes happen, so a responsible cook should know what to do when a friend eats too many milligrams (page 45). But keeping the dose low allows people to find their tolerance without the long-term commitment of a more potent edible.

A Formula for an Ethical Dose

When I started cooking with weed, my idea of how much to put in a recipe followed the logic of Italian nonnas: "Quanto basta," however much is enough. Except this wasn't flour, and I wasn't making pasta. The consequence of adding too much hash meant the difference between a leisurely, sparkly-eyed afternoon and the walls melting around me. Using experimentation first, then science, I created a formula that allows you to confidently eat your heart out.

The dose of any edible stems from the potency of whatever flower or concentrate the recipe calls for. Average potencies of flower and concentrates vary as much as the alcohol content in wines. Trim usually tests anywhere from 15 to 25 percent THCA. I've seen indoor flower boasting over 35 percent THCA potency. Concentrates, such as hash and kief, range from 50 to up to 80 percent THCA, rosins reach higher than 80 percent, and distillates from crude, full-spectrum oils come in as high as 90 percent. Further purified isolates reach nearly 100 percent THC.

This book calculates dosage based on 25 percent THCA flower, but every recipe inevitably involves some loss of potency. From the decarboxylation process to the streaks of infused cake batter left inside the bowl, expect to lose anywhere from 15 to 20 percent of the THCA potency labeled. The 25 percent THCA flower with the standard 12.3 percent loss of potency after decarboxylation, minus an additional 7.7 percent for cooking mishaps, becomes 20 percent THC. That is the base I use for calculating doses in written recipes.

I calculate the doses in both the Mother Infusions and the individual recipes in this book—meaning you can skip the math if you start with 25 percent THCA flower. You can also skip it if you use a distillate concentrate, which has already been decarboxylated (see Cooking with Concentrates, page 33). But everyone from a casual cannabis cook to a professional pot pastry producer should know how to figure out the general strength of their snacks, and these steps simplify the process.

How to Calculate the Strength of an Infusion:

(THCA in milligrams x 0.8) x **PLF** = **P** (Potency)

(**P** x grams of flower used in infusion)
÷ yield of infusion in tablespoons
= **I** (Infusion strength)

READ THE LABEL: Regulated weed comes with a label listing the cannabinoid content of the flower or concentrate. Look for the THC percentage, which is, technically, THCA for flower or raw concentrates. Twenty-five percent THCA means the flower contains 250 milligrams of THCA per gram.

Infusion Formulas

Multiply the total milligrams by
the potency loss factor (plf)

Mother Infusion	Potency Loss Factor (PLF)	Leftover Potency
Cannabutter	1	N/A
Brown Cannabutter	1	N/A
Oils	1	N/A
Milks	0.5	50%
120 Proof Tincture	0.4	60%
Frozen 120 Proof Tincture	0.2	80%

TO CALCULATE LOSS FROM DECARBOXYLATION AND COOKING: Multiply the milligrams of THCA by 0.8 to calculate the 20 percent loss (explained above).

TO CALCULATE ADDITIONAL POTENCY LOSS FACTOR: Different infusions extract different percentages of THC, so the number of milligrams needs to be multiplied by percent of potency for that infusion. The Cannabutters (pages 61–62) and OOO Oil (page 64) infuse nearly 100 percent of the THC, so this step can be skipped, as they would be multiplied by 1. For any other infusion, multiply by the potency loss factor (PLF) shown in the chart below.

SCALE UP: The figure P is in milligrams per gram, so to scale up your infusion, multiply P by the number of grams used in the infusion recipe and divide by the number of tablespoons in the total quantity to get I, the strength of your infusion per tablespoon.

SAMPLE CALCULATION: If I were to use 28 percent THCA flower to create a 120-proof (room temperature) tincture, I would use the following calculation: (280 x .8) x .4 = 89.6 milligrams THC per gram of flower used. This is the number P that I use below to calculate the amount needed to dose an edible recipe.

Since the tincture recipe in this book uses 6 grams of weed, to scale up, I multiply 90 milligrams THC by 6, making the entire batch 540 milligrams of THC, or 67.5 milligrams of THC per tablespoon.

How to Calculate the Dose of an Edible:

Servings x 5 milligrams = **T** (Total milligrams THC needed)

T ÷ (**P** or **I**) = Total quantity needed for a recipe of decarboxylated weed in grams (if **P**) or tablespoons of infusion (if **I**).

ESTIMATE SERVINGS: Look at the recipe and consider the real-life situation to estimate how many servings someone will truly eat, factoring in the time of day and how much other food will be around. Then assume most people will eat more than you think.

CALCULATE TOTAL THC NEEDED: Five milligrams per serving is an ideal dose; use that to calculate the potency needed for a batch. Multiply the estimated number of servings in the batch by 5. I call this number T, the total milligrams THC needed to make the recipe.

CALCULATE THE TOTAL FLOWER OR INFUSION NEEDED: If you are adding the decarboxylated flower directly to the recipe: Divide T (total milligrams THC needed to make the recipe) by P (power in milligrams per gram) to get the total amount of flower, in grams, of decarboxylated weed needed for your recipe.

IF YOU ARE ADDING AN INFUSION: Divide T (total milligrams THC to dose the recipe) by I (power in milligrams per tablespoon) to get the amount of Cannabutter, Mota Milk, OOO Oil, or any other Mother Infusion needed for the recipe.

SAMPLE CALCULATION: With the Peach Dreamsicles (page 204), a batch makes 10 frozen treats, or 10 servings. Dessert comes last, so I want to keep these at 3 milligrams each, meaning 30 total milligrams of THC. The recipe calls for a room-temperature tincture infusion, so using the one we calculated above, which has an I of 67.5 milligrams per tablespoon, we divide the T (30) by the I (67.5) and get that we need 0.44 tablespoons, or a scant half tablespoon, of tincture.

HOW TO ADJUST A RECIPE FOR A DIFFERENT DOSE: Sometimes you will need to alter the recipe to account for the potency of flower, concentrate, or infusion. To lessen it, simply substitute the necessary quantity of infused for un-infused oil, butter, or whatever ingredient holds the power. To make a dish stronger, you will need to use a stronger infusion. In the case of the dreamsicles, to make them lighter, I simply use less tincture. To make them stronger, I would infuse more flower in the Turnt Tincture (page 70) to start, since adding more alcohol to the recipe will alter the dreamsicle.

HOW TO STORE EDIBLES

Neglecting to label a batch of dosed cookies and sticking them in a random container in the freezer signs everyone up for a round of edible roulette, a game that people rarely win. Save your future self, houseguests, or others from an accidental bad trip by labeling edibles as if lives depend on it.

It merits repeating: Always clearly and loudly mark homemade edibles. Hungry people skip over words like *special* or *magical*, choosing to interpret them as synonyms for delicious, even though we know them as euphemisms. Spell it out in bold letters for people—THIS CONTAINS WEED—and note roughly how many milligrams per serving (included with each recipe in this book). I've gotten too many frantic phone calls from friends who never thought to label the edibles they'd hidden on the top shelf that someone got into.

When Swedish singer Lykke Li came on *Bong Appétit*, she shared a childhood memory from when her parents left a plate of weed cookies out on the counter and she ate several before they noticed. The hours of disorientation as a kid ensured that, as a parent, she takes extra precautions to avoid risking her own children doing the same. When kids live in the house, treat edibles like medicine. Store-bought edibles must come in child-resistant (and often stoner-resistant) packaging. Follow the same principles with homemade versions, ideally keeping them in a locking canister. Opaque containers ensure jars of tantalizing weed cookies stay hidden from sugar-seeking munchkins. Take even more precaution than you might with alcohol: While alcohol tastes gross, dosed treats taste pretty close to the original—but with traumatizing effects for kids.

WHEN SOMEONE GETS TOO HIGH

First and foremost, stay calm: They are likely going to be just fine on their own, but it can still *feel* horrific for whoever ate too many bites of brownie, so do your best to make them feel safe. If that means alone, tucked in bed, watching *How High*, and munching on a peanut butter banana sandwich, then make it happen.

A friend who's totally zonked on weed is having what's known as a green out, and they will thank you later for guiding them through it. If it seems like a medical emergency, the best thing to do is call 911.

Getting my weed chocolates to Puglia, in Italy's south, involved a half-pound box of See's Candies, shrink wrap, and expert sticker removal. Hanging out by the pool of the rustic Italian farmhouse the day before my wedding, my cousin from Rome wanted to try an edible for the first time. I agreed but told her to eat only a quarter of a chocolate and see how she felt. She did. Then she ate a little bit more.

An hour later, she came up to me with her makeup smeared all over her face—she had splashed herself with water in an effort to stop feeling so stoned. It failed.

I explained that the effects would wear off after a few hours, and that edibles hit differently than smoking. She kept checking her pulse to make sure she still had a heartbeat. After I calmed her down and explained again that she would not and could not die, I went to finish arranging the reception seating chart. But 30 minutes later, I spotted the red lights of an ambulance as they lit up the olive trees lining the driveway to our rented farmhouse.

After several hours of surveillance at the hospital, my cousin returned, feeling embarrassed. I reassured her that she wasn't the first person to have a bad trip on edibles—after all, even the doctors in that small town in Puglia had enough experience to know that the only true remedy was waiting it out.

Weddings magnify stress, and my zio's concern about his daughter having a heart attack only escalated my cousin's anxiety. Even though I knew she would be okay, my family did the right thing: If someone insists on going to the hospital, take them. Having a doctor say they won't die holds a lot more weight than their stoner cousin from California saying the same thing.

But, if things are under control, before calling the paramedics, there are a few anecdotal remedies you might try first.

Some word-of-mouth methods tap into the terpenes found in other foods to counteract effects of THC. Cannabis users have long touted the quick remedy of a lemon peel or rosemary tea for their uplifting benefits. They claim the limonene found in citrus and pinene in rosemary will counteract the high. On the other hand, the myrcene found in mangoes is said to make a high feel heavier, so maybe leave it alone.

There is another method for mitigating a potent cannabis high that actually has some scientific research to back it up, and it conveniently uses something most people probably have on hand in the moment of crisis. Beta-caryophyllene, found in black pepper, cloves, and other spices, is a very special terpene because it's also a phytocannabinoid. It binds to the same cannabinoid receptors (CB2) as THC, potentially replacing the THC. While CB2 receptors have little effect on the psychoactivity of weed, chewing on black peppercorns supposedly has a calming effect.

Studies have yet to prove whether any of these work. But a plate of cacio e pepe with a few extra grinds of black pepper definitely cures the munchies. And if it potentially mellows the high, too, I'll eat my placebos in pasta form, grazie.

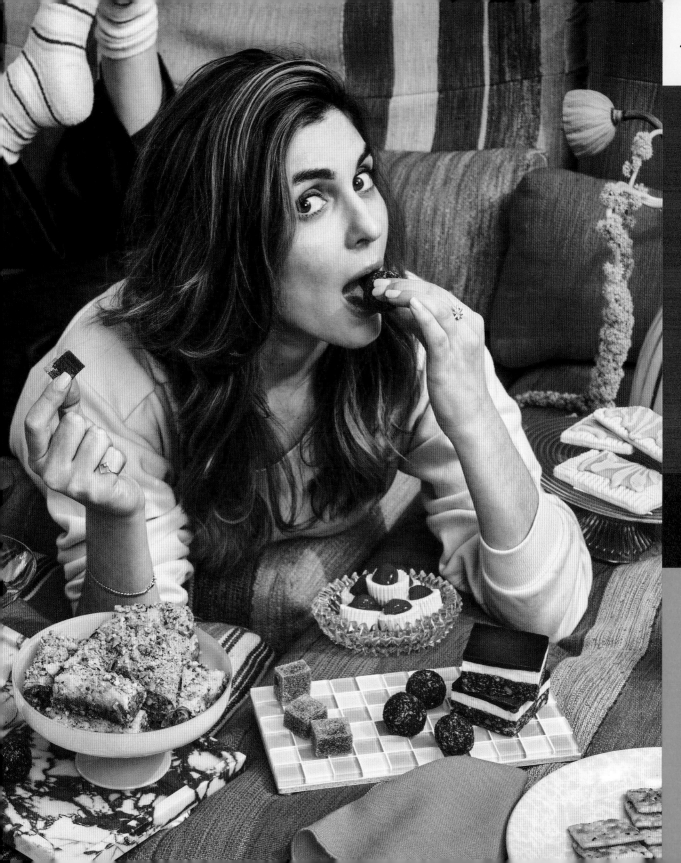

How to Eat Weed & Have a Good Time

Homogeneity and the Last Bowl of Chicken Soup

One time back in my experimental era, I felt under the weather and was curious about whether I could decarb raw hash directly into my chicken soup. I added a pinch of hash to my mirepoix, sizzling in schmaltz in the bottom of a Dutch oven. It seemed a miniscule amount for an entire pot of soup, and I doubted the THCA would even convert to THC. I never considered what happens to the seasoned schmaltz in soup.

The difference between a good time and an accidental bad trip boils down to the proper distribution of a dose. Imagine chunks of decarboxylated hash haphazardly sprinkled onto a batch of toffee as it cools: Some portions of candy get speckled with huge resin goobers and others are left with mere crumbs. When someone breaks off a piece with more hash, they'll soar, while someone else might think they got ripped off because they feel nothing. To avoid that happening, the dose needs to be evenly distributed. In the case of a toffee, whisking the hash into melted butter before adding the mixture to the hot candy spreads the dose throughout the confection. In the case of chicken soup, it took me to the last spoonful to find out that the hash did, in fact, decarb, and that emulsifying the dose is an essential part of cooking weed.

I shared a bowl of soup with a friend visiting from out of town who kept lamenting how stressed out she felt. I figured a bit of hash chicken soup might help. We both slurped up the soothing broth, then waited to feel the effects. The soup gave us a slight tingle, but hardly the high we expected. I assumed my experiment failed.

The next day, my friend devoured the final bowl of the presumably benign soup for lunch, scooping every last drop into her bowl—and unknowingly eating the majority of the dose. All the cannabinoids stuck to the schmaltz, which floated to the top of the soup and stuck to the sides of the pot. She had a few words for me, once she could talk straight.

THC naturally gravitates toward fat. Since the chicken soup consisted mostly of water, the dose concentrated in the tiny proportion of schmaltz in the soup. Had I made a cream of chicken soup, where the fat blends throughout the pot, the dose would have been administered more evenly. Instead, my friend got smacked in the face by a heady schmaltz.

Getting creative with dosing is fun, but ensuring homogeneity throughout a dish is essential. When I make Marigold Sweets salted caramels, rather than throwing the concentrate directly into the caramel, I whisk it thoroughly into melted butter before adding it to the batch. Commercial enterprises often employ lecithin, which helps emulsify fats with liquids and thus distributes the dose evenly. Lecithin also makes baked goods more shelf stable through a freeze-thaw cycle, which matters a lot when distributing.

On *Bong Appétit*, we tried to maximize the number of infusions in one dish, because the show aimed to demonstrate the versatility of weed as an ingredient. At home, I infuse only one element of a recipe because then there are fewer variables to control in order to dose. For example, in cupcakes, both the frosting and the cake contain an easily infusible fat. But if I infuse the frosting, I have to make sure every cupcake gets the same amount of frosting, and my piping skills lack the consistency to execute that. With an infused cake batter, I can easily scoop or weigh out the same amount into every paper cup. The scale never lies, and nobody wants their trip to be captained by a stoner trying to squeeze frosting into the shape of a rose.

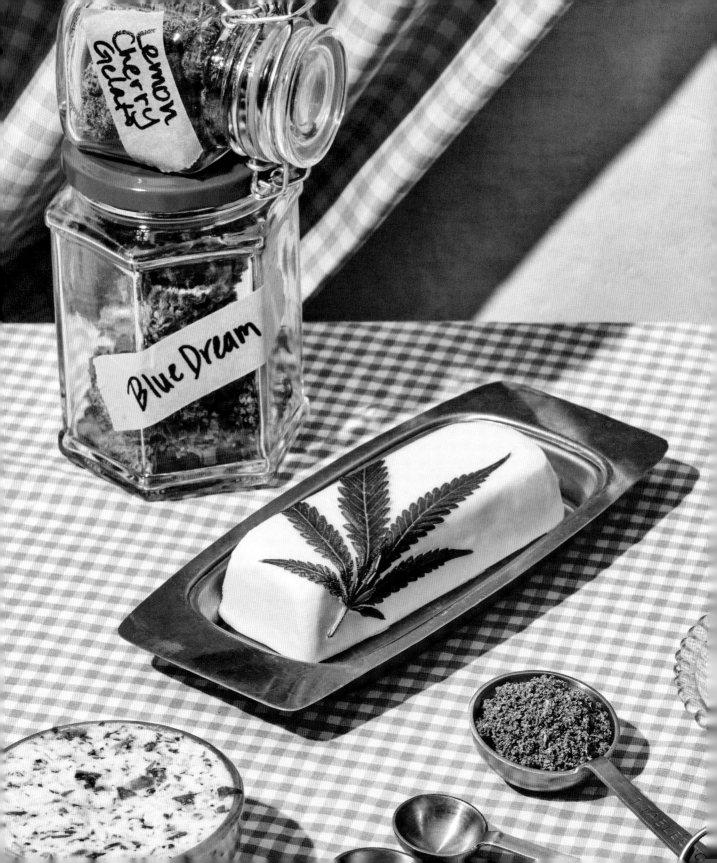

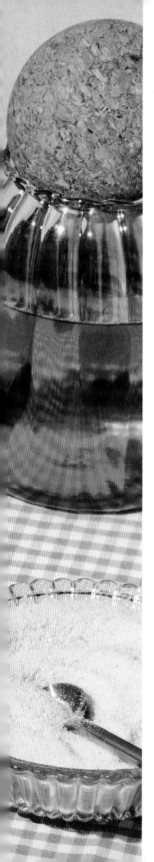

HOW TO COOK WEED

The best way to enjoy eating weed is to cook with it. Easily digestible, lightly dosed, and fun-to-eat recipes make the best edibles. A giant plate of super-chronic weed lasagna sounds like a great idea, but after hours of paralytic couch lock, you won't be going back for seconds. And that would make my nonna very sad.

With everything from cooking essentials to gifts that get you geeked, this book shows the versatility of cannabis as an ingredient. Each of the recipes, including hors d'oeuvres, side dishes, snacks, drinks, baked goods, sweets, and goody bags, offers a lightly dosed portion. For high-tolerance folks, serving suggestions show how to combine dishes for a heavier hit.

Start with a super-simple snack, then try your hand at one of the complicated, delicate pastries—which may require a sober supervisor (look for the "Heads up, Pothead!" warnings). From there, plan a menu and invite friends to partake at your pot party. Let's roll!

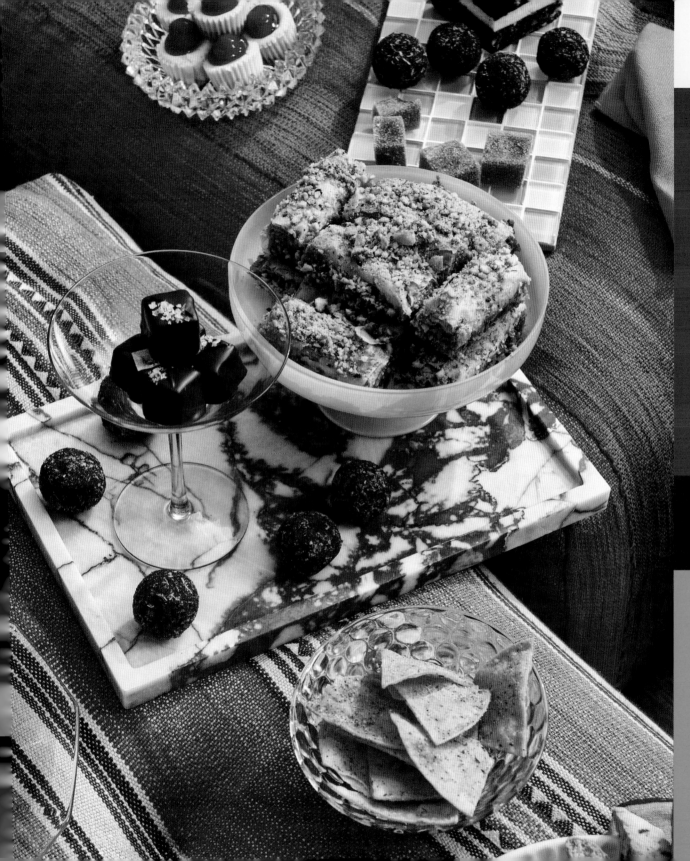

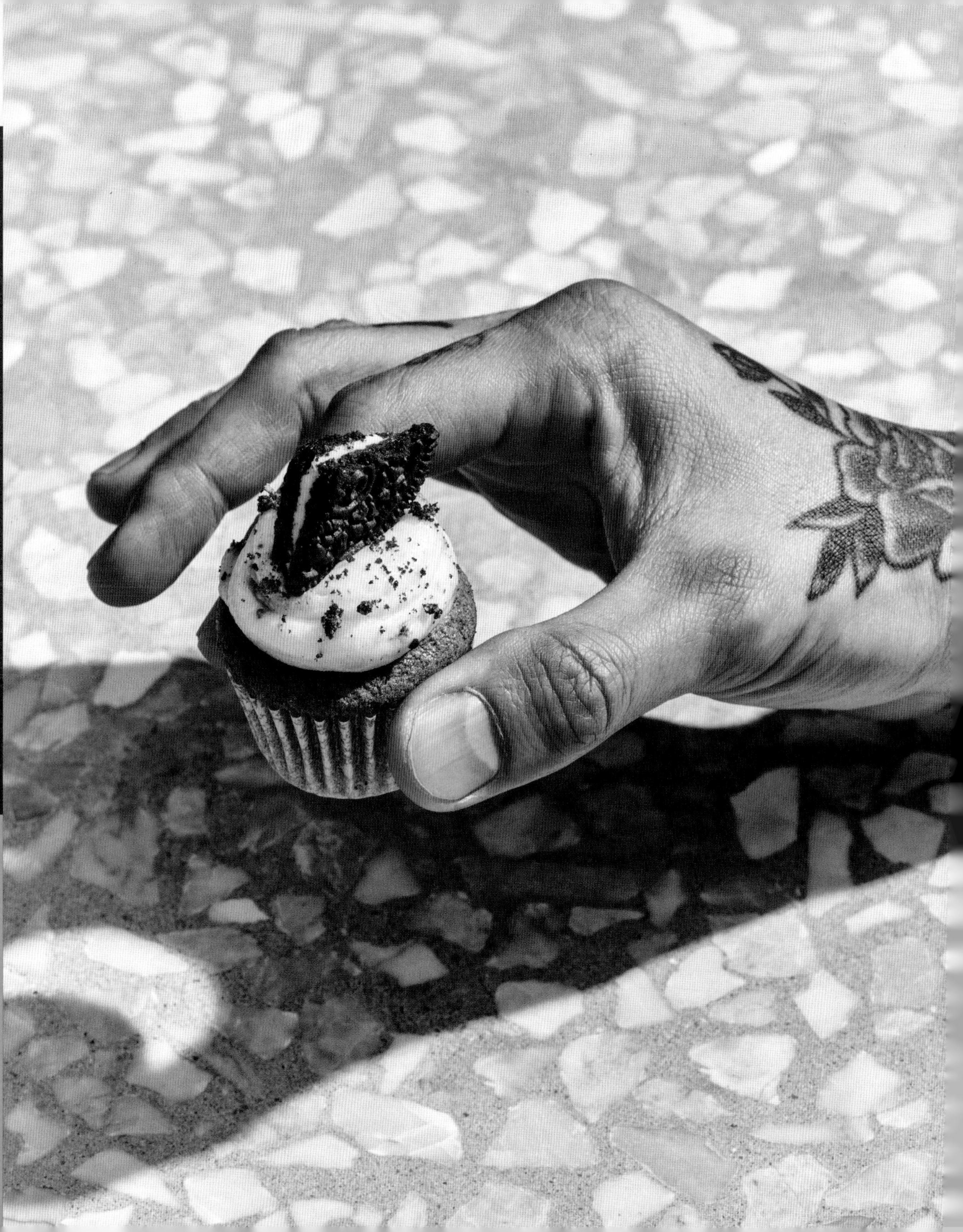

THE POT PANTRY

The secret to cooking well with cannabis lies in a well-stocked kitchen. This chapter dives deep into my Mother Infusions of Cannabutter, OOO Oil, Mota Milk, and Turnt Tinctures. They work in recipes in this book and beyond, so your next high is never out of arm's reach.

MOTHER INFUSIONS

My Sicilian grandfather instructed me to believe none of what I hear, and only half of what I see. Grandpa Ned's advice turns out to apply doubly to cannabis information, as I learned when I started running experiments at a lab in 2020. The results blew away the infusion rates found in recipes, many of which called for multiple hours sweating over the stove; my Brown Cannabutter (page 62) reached full infusion within 10 minutes.

The data I collected through more than two hundred experiments on different fats, milks, and alcohols shows how efficiently cannabinoids infuse, especially into fats. The results informed the techniques used in this book, especially the Mother Infusions in this section: base batches of butters, oils, milks, and alcohols designed to maximize potency, minimize time, and prioritize flavor. Each of the Mother Infusion recipes can be extrapolated to a category of cannabis infusions, then kept on hand to add doses quickly and easily to any dish—and do so in most of the recipes in this book.

In two decades as a pothead, I have listened to amateurs and experts alike emphasize the importance of steeping weed in butter for hours on end, because more time means greater potency. A stoned starlet at a New York City nightclub once told me weed butter reaches full potency only after twelve hours of constant stirring under a full moon. It sounds wild, but a more reliable source, *High Times*, still suggests a whopping six-hour method,

though without the astrological requirement. Most tincture recipes subscribe to the same theory to infuse alcohol. The first time I attempted a tincture, I followed instructions that required a two-month infusion in the freezer. My lab tests found that the exaggerated infusion time failed to produce a substantially improved tincture.

On top of saving precious time, shorter infusions extract fewer of the unsavory plant compounds, resulting in better flavor and lighter color. In an 1866 candy cookbook I have, *The Art of Confectionery*, the author quotes a Chinese saying: "We injure tea by letting water stand too long upon it." The same can be said about cannabutter or any other infusion. Over-steeping the weed creates a bitter flavor, with little impact on the potency.

To avoid that, I searched for ways to speed up the process and found that temperature matters most in how quickly the cannabinoids infuse, while agitation (usually by stirring) also accelerates the separation of trichomes (the cannabinoid-packed glands of the plant) from the plant material.

Through my many experiments, I found a sweet spot for the maximum infusion of cannabinoids without compromising on flavor. The four Mother Infusions in this chapter are the optimized recipes for infusing butter, oil, milk, and alcohol with weed, getting your pot pantry off to a quick start and preparing you to make many of the recipes that follow.

CANNABUTTER

Cannabutter has long been the classic infusion used in cannabis cooking, and for good reason: Fat carries the flavor of food, and the high, too. When we cook with weed, THC easily dissolves into any fat, and when we eat weed, fat helps our bodies to metabolize the THC.

Out of the five different fats I infused and lab tested, butter infused the fastest at the lowest temperature, with 60 percent of the THC infusing into the butter after just 30 seconds at 190ºF, and 83 percent after 10 minutes.

Unlike a pure oil, butter is an emulsion of water, milk proteins, and butterfat, and the combination makes a powerful solvent for weed. It works so well that currently used infusion times are excessive. After one hour at 190ºF, butter starts to get weird and fails miserably at what is known in food science as an organoleptic evaluation: It looks and tastes terrible. At 30 minutes, nearly 100 percent of the THC infuses into the butter;

cooking it any longer wastes time and degrades taste.

The other common mistake with cannabutter comes when the infusion process messes with the texture of the butter, resulting in a grainy product rather than a silky smooth spread. Thankfully, my experience with chocolate has taught me a thing or two about melting stable emulsions. When we heat butter, like when we heat chocolate, the heat breaks the emulsion and changes the balance of ingredients. Think of how microwaved butter gets after cooling in the fridge: It separates into layers and the texture gets grainy.

To re-emulsify the finished cannabutter, I infuse half of the butter in a double boiler for 30 minutes. I remove it from the heat and stir in cold butter to bring the emulsion back together, much like the process of tempering chocolate. As the cold butter slowly melts, it blends the milk solids, water, and infused butterfat back together into a

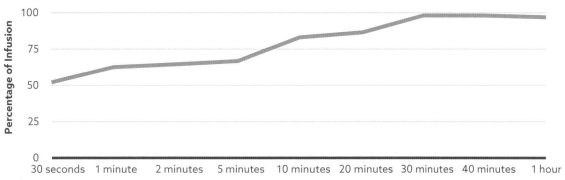

Butter Infusion Rate 190°F

56 grams (1/4 cup) of butter infused with 3 grams (18% THC) flower

strong, smooth emulsion that cools as a solid mass rather than separated layers.

All the recipes in this book that call for cannabutter use 2 grams of decarboxylated flower in 1 cup of butter. People use too much weed when they cook! This cannabutter and other infusions in this book focus on flavor and serving size, so people can eat more than one bite. I know that many home edible makers prefer to make a large batch of highly potent cannabutter. If that applies to you, use the chart below to calculate roughly how many milligrams of THC end up in a tablespoon of butter based on the amount of flower added to the butter. The potency of the flower will change the potency of the butter, but this gives a general idea about the ratio of flower to butter. If you make a stronger butter, you can add regular butter to dilute the potency and avoid hyper-dosing the recipes in the book that call for cannabutter. Find more information on dosing in A Formula for an Ethical Dose (page 42).

Decarboxylated Flower (20% THC) in 1 Cup Butter

1 gram	2 grams	3.5 grams	7 grams	14 grams
12.5 mg	25 mg	43.75 mg	87.5 mg	175 mg

mg THC per tablespoon butter

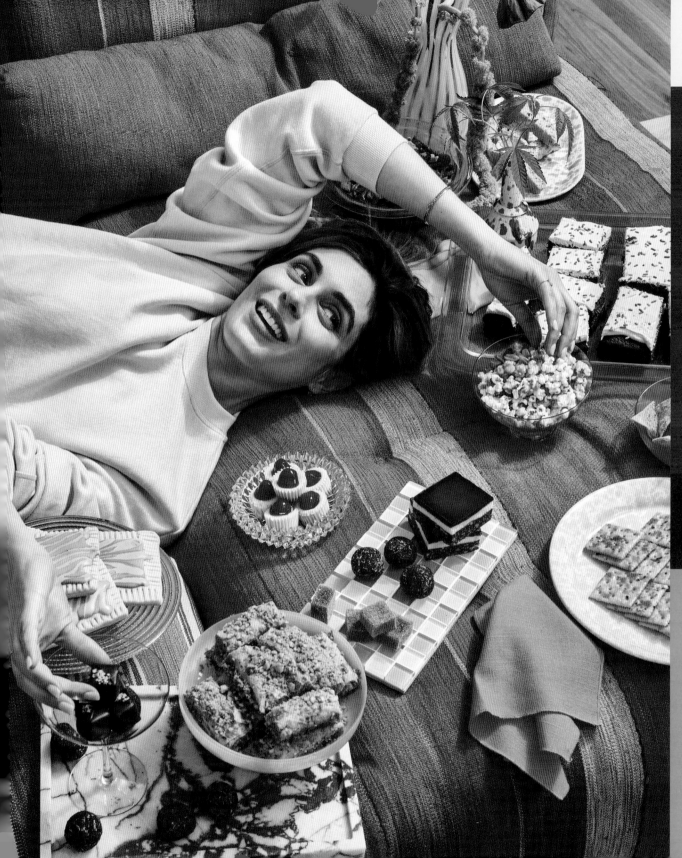

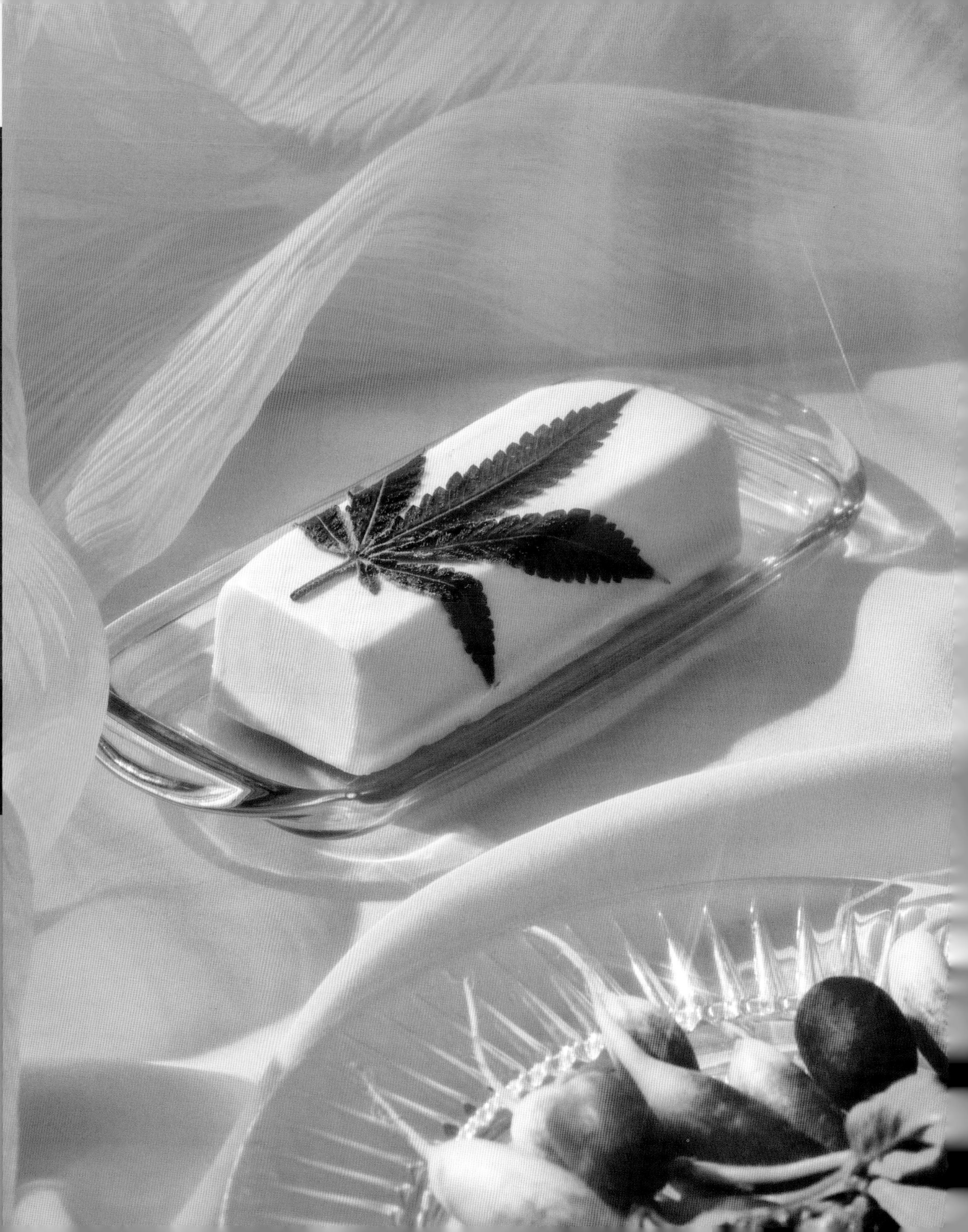

CANNABUTTER

MAKES 1 cup

TIME: 50 minutes

DOSE: 25 mg THC
per tablespoon

1 / Make a double boiler by filling a 3-quart saucepan with 2 cups of water and placing a medium metal bowl on top. Set the double boiler over low heat and add ½ cup of the unsalted butter to the bowl. When it fully melts and reaches 190°F, 4 to 5 minutes, add the 2 tablespoons of water and the flower. Vigorously whisk everything together for 15 seconds, then cover the bowl with a lid, so the steam condenses and drips back into the fat. Continue whisking vigorously for 15 seconds every 5 minutes, for a total of 30 minutes.

2 / Remove the bowl from the heat and pour the butter through a cheesecloth-lined strainer into another medium bowl. Wait for the flower to cool enough to touch, 1 to 2 minutes, then gather the cheesecloth and wring out every last drop of butter from it. Let the butter cool for a few more minutes, then use a rubber spatula to stir the remaining ½ cup of cold butter cubes into the infused butter until they melt together into a single creamy mass. Pour into an airtight lidded container to store in the fridge for up to 3 weeks, or measure out tablespoon portions into ice cube trays, freeze, then pop them out into a freezer bag and put back into the freezer for up to 3 months.

1 cup (8 ounces) cold unsalted butter, cubed, divided

2 tablespoons water

2 grams ground decarboxylated flower

BROWN CANNABUTTER

MAKES ⅓ cup

TIME: 15 minutes

DOSE: 100 mg THC
per ⅓ cup

While my Cannabutter recipe already speeds up the traditional infusion process, this recipe takes it even further, combining two of my favorite things in the world: shortcuts and brown butter. An easy way to speed up an infusion is to raise the temperature of the solvent. But, in standard cannabutter infusions, the water content of butter ensures that the temperature remains under 212°F, the boiling point of water. That limits how quickly the infusion can happen and dictates the minimum speed.

Enter brown butter, which boils off the water while simultaneously caramelizing the milk solids and infusing the THC into the fat. In the 10 minutes it takes for the butter to brown, the THC binds to the fat. Plus, the nutty caramel notes hide the pot flavor in sweeter recipes, such as the Fudgy Fluffernutty Brownies (page 166).

1 / In a small saucepan, combine the butter and flower and set over medium-low heat. Use a rubber spatula to stir constantly, to keep the bottom from scorching, especially as the butter foams up. When the foam subsides and the milk solids begin to brown, 8 to 10 minutes, remove the pan from the heat. Pour the butter through a cheesecloth-lined strainer into a small bowl.

2 / Wait a few minutes for the flower to cool, then gather the cheesecloth and squeeze out any excess butter from the flower. Use immediately or store in an airtight container and keep refrigerated for up to 2 weeks, or freeze for up to 3 months.

½ cup (4 ounces) unsalted butter
½ gram ground decarboxylated flower

OIL

Olive oil reigns in my house: Because I use it to make salad dressings, thicken hummus, and cook down peppers for peperonata, among many other applications, I focused my experiments on creating the ideal infused olive oil—and it turned out to work across all types of oil, from canola to coconut.

As noted in the Brown Cannabutter recipe, heating speeds up infusion, and unlike butter, oil has no water to worry about. The only concern is keeping it under any temperature that will either fry the weed or degrade the oil. Heating oil to 240°F, well below the smoking point of any oil, is plenty hot to partially infuse in a matter of minutes, and in 20 minutes, the majority of the THC will have infused.

Percentage of Infusion at 190°F

Type of Fat	5 Minutes	10 Minutes	20 Minutes	40 Minutes
Butter	66%	83%	86%	98%
Olive Oil	63%	66%	70%	73%
Coconut Oil	50%	52%	70%	72%
Vegetable Oil	50%	54%	62%	70%
Grapeseed Oil	45%	52%	57%	61%

OOO OIL

MAKES 1 cup

TIME: 35 minutes

DOSE: 25 mg THC
per tablespoon

This recipe works with any oil. Throughout the book, I refer to this with whichever type of oil is used in the recipe: OOO Olive Oil, OOO Coconut Oil, etc.

1 / Preheat the oven to 240°F.

2 / In a large, oven-safe ramekin, bake the oil for 10 minutes, then check that the oil is 240°F before continuing. Use a small whisk to vigorously stir the flower into the heated oil. Leave it in the oven for 20 more minutes, stirring every 5 minutes, then pour the infused oil through a cheesecloth-lined strainer into a bowl. Let the flower cool for a few minutes, then gather the cheesecloth and squeeze out the last drops of infused oil.

3 / Store the oil in the refrigerator, as the added plant material makes it go rancid more easily. It should last 1 to 2 months, or you can keep it in the freezer for up to 4 months. Remember to label it.

1 cup oil, any type

2 grams ground decarboxylated flower

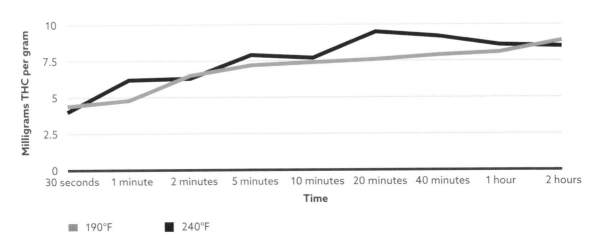

Olive Oil Infusion Rate

56 grams (¼ cup) of olive oil infused with 3 grams (18% THC) flower

Milligrams THC per gram — Time: 30 seconds, 1 minute, 2 minutes, 5 minutes, 10 minutes, 20 minutes, 40 minutes, 1 hour, 2 hours

■ 190°F   ■ 240°F

MILK

When I cooked with my edible maker friend Ice in her kitchen outside Bangkok, she mentioned that infused milk takes on a more bitter flavor from the weed than butter or oil. When it comes to infusion, the main question to ask is: Got fat? While milk contains fat, it also contains water, which extracts the bitter compounds, along with the potency, from the weed. That means infused milk can have a green flavor you might not want in a bowl of breakfast cereal. As long as the infused milk acts as a backup singer in a recipe rather than the lead vocalist, the flavors will harmonize.

As with tea, the longer plants sit in a hot liquid, the more bitter the flavor becomes. I found that it took one hour of infusion for whole milk to extract nearly all the available THC from flower, but the result smelled a lot like a garbage bag full of old trim left to sit out in the sun for too long. In my attempt to create an appetizing milk, I found that the flavor turned after 10 minutes. According to my lab tests, the short infusion pulls 50 percent of the potency from the weed and leaves no musty aftertaste. That leaves half of the high in the flower, which would break my heart, so I created the recipe for Herbaceous Meatballs (page 96) with this lower-dose leftover flower. My nonna would be proud—waste not, want not.

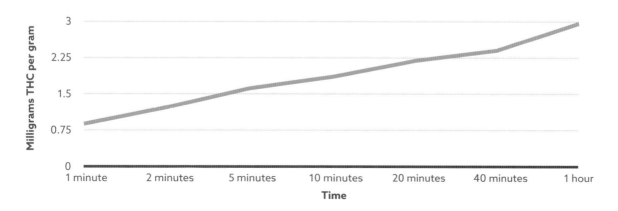

Whole Milk Infusion Rate 190°F

200 grams of whole milk infused with 4 grams (18% THC) flower

Milligrams THC per gram

3
2.25
1.5
0.75
0

1 minute — 2 minutes — 5 minutes — 10 minutes — 20 minutes — 40 minutes — 1 hour

Time

MOTA MILK

MAKES 1 cup

TIME: 15 minutes

DOSE: 6.25 mg THC
per tablespoon

As with the oil, this recipe can be used for a variety of milks, including dairy and coconut, but depending on the fat content of the milk (e.g., cashew is high fat), the potency may vary. If you use a higher fat milk or cream, you'll extract more THC. I ran tests on infusions of coconut and whole (cow's) milk and can verify the potency results; thus, those are the two varieties used in this book.

1 / In a 2-quart saucepan, warm the milk on low heat to just below a simmer. Add the flower and whisk every minute for a total of 10 minutes. Pour the milk through a cheesecloth-lined strainer into a cup or jar. Let the flower cool for a few minutes, then gather the cheesecloth and squeeze out the remaining milk.

2 / Use the milk right away or store in a labeled airtight container in the fridge for 1 to 2 days. To store it for up to 2 months, freeze in an ice cube tray and pop the milk cubes out into a bag labeled with the dose per cube or tablespoon. Use the leftover flower in the Herbaceous Meatballs (page 96).

1 cup whole milk or coconut milk (or any other milk with similar fat content)

1 gram decarboxylated ground flower

ALCOHOL

Infusing weed into alcohol makes a versatile liquid extract of THC called a tincture. When a recipe calls for an oil, butter, or other fat, I see an opportunity to infuse weed. When I come across a recipe without a fatty entryway, I turn to an alcohol tincture. Unfortunately, since cannabinoids prefer fat, the infusion of alcohol is less effective than oils or butters.

Anyone who has cleaned a bong before knows the higher the proof (or stronger the rubbing alcohol), the more easily the torched resin comes off. The same goes for making tincture. As with the fats, most existing recipes assumed a longer infusion time produced a more potent tincture, but, once again, my lab testing proved that wrong. The data made it clear that alcohol proof, rather than time, dictates the infusion rate of cannabinoids into alcohol. A higher proof and a swift whisk result in a more potent infusion than a longer steep, and a majority of the infusion happens in the first 30 seconds.

Whether working with 120-proof or 190-proof alcohol, the percentage of cannabinoids infused generally plateaus within 15 minutes of whisking the flower into the alcohol. For 120-proof, 40 percent infuses into the alcohol, whereas 190-proof extracts 70 percent. The recipes in this book use a 120-proof tincture, mainly because it is the highest widely accessible proof across the country (and because California changed the laws right before I started writing this book and the grocery store selling bootleg booze got caught).

The lower the proof of a spirit, the more water and less ethanol available to extract cannabinoids, and the water also pulls other unsavory flavors from the plant. Commercial concentrate producers use pure ethanol and extreme temperatures to avoid this issue.

As with the fat-based infusion, temperature comes into play with alcohol as the solvent. To prevent the tincture from turning a sludgy green, keep

Alcohol Infusion by Proof

60 ml of alcohol infused with 3 grams (18% THC) flower for 10 minutes at room temperature

Alcohol Proof	80	120	190
Milligrams THC per milliliter of tincture	0.5 mg	4 mg	7 mg
Milligrams THC per tablespoon of tincture	7.5 mg	60 mg	105 mg

the solvent ice cold. When making cold-water hash, the hash maker uses ice water to chill the trichome heads so they break off and fall through fine micron screens, separated from the larger plant matter. Likewise, putting the alcohol in the freezer before adding the decarboxylated flower keeps the plant's chlorophyll from absorbing into the tincture, making a clearer product. But it also affects the potency: While a freezer-made tincture improves the flavor tenfold, it decreases the potency by 50 percent.

I ran a battery of tests in search of the ideal tincture technique. I made tinctures that sat at room temperature for a month and turned into powerful swamps, and I used nitrous oxide, applied via whipped cream canister, to turbo-charge others. Each time the lab results came back the same: The only methods that increased potency failed taste tests, and the nitrous did nothing at all.

I found that the easiest and fastest way to make a potent and palatable tincture takes just 15 minutes and a little stirring. For recipes where other ingredients will mask the flavor, I use the room temperature tincture recipe. When the flavor of the tincture stands front and center, like in the Marshmellows (page 215), I use a similar method, with a longer infusion time for a freezer tincture (see instructions below the recipe). In this book, when I call for tincture without otherwise specifying, I'm referring to the standard room temperature version, so adjust for quantity and dosing if using freezer-made tincture.

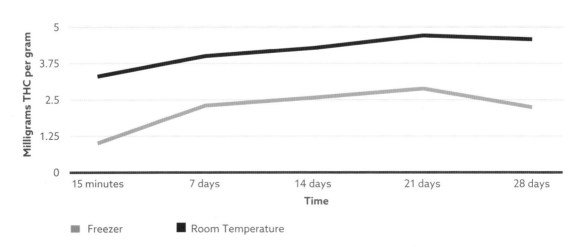

120-Proof Tincture Infusion Rate

100 grams of alcohol infused with 6 grams (18% THC) flower

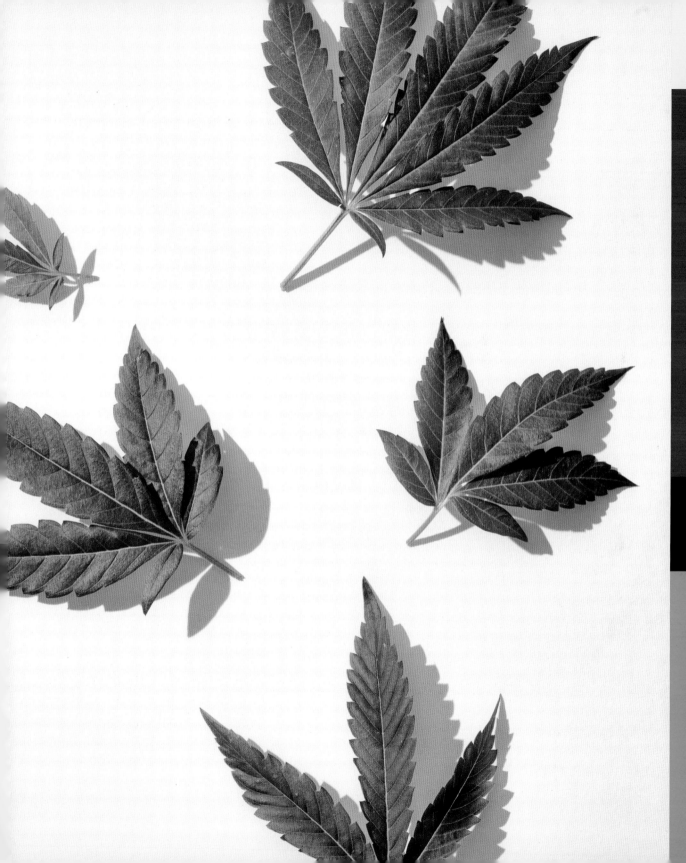

TURNT TINCTURE

MAKES ½ cup

TIME: 15 minutes
(plus 1 week, for
frozen tincture)

DOSE: 60 mg THC
per tablespoon
(30 mg THC per
tablespoon freezer
tincture)

1 / In a medium bowl, whisk together the alcohol and flower for 30 seconds, then whisk vigorously every 2 minutes for a total of 10 minutes. Pour through a cheesecloth-lined strainer into a jar. Squeeze any remaining liquid from the flower in the cheesecloth.

2 / Store the tincture in a labeled airtight container in the freezer for up to a month.

3 / Alternative method: To make a freezer-made tincture, start with ice-cold alcohol. After whisking, leave it in a jar in the freezer to infuse for up to three weeks, giving the jar a shake every day. Strain and store as instructed above.

½ cup 120-proof neutral grain alcohol

6 grams ground decarboxylated flower

Reduce, Reuse, Rehash

After making room temperature Turnt Tincture, the alcohol-soaked flower will still contain 60 percent of its original potency, or 720 milligrams of THC per batch. If it's freezer-made Turnt Tincture, the flower will retain 80 percent of its original potency. To dry it out for use as a lower-potency strain, preheat the oven to 180°F and spread the flower out on a parchment-paper-lined sheet pan. Bake for 30 to 40 minutes, until the flower feels dry to the touch. Weigh the flower and divide 720 milligrams by the total mass to calculate the milligrams per gram of flower, then use it to cook.

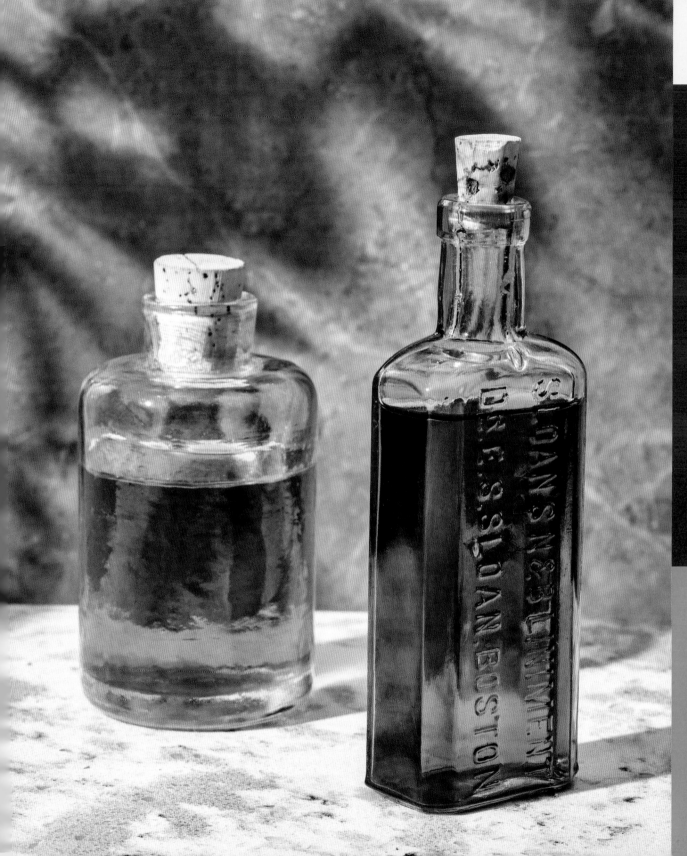

Accidentally Dosing My Ex: A Lesson on Cannabis Cross-Contamination

One lazy Saturday, I infused a batch of cinnamon toffee with CO_2 distillate and used a paring knife to scrape it into the pot. I left the knife next to the sink, with every intention to wash it, eventually. Unfortunately, my ex got hungry before I did.

He sauntered into the kitchen, picked up the dirty paring knife on the counter to slice cheese, layered the cheddar with several pieces of ham, griddled it between hunks of crusty bread, and dug in. After lunch, per Italian custom, he took a nap on the couch.

Thirty minutes later, as I packaged a fresh batch of Marigold Sweets at the dining table, he yelled from the living room, "Vané, I feel high." At first, he blamed it on secondhand smoke from my joint, but I knew that made zero sense: While a contact high is possible with extreme exposure, nobody trips from the smoke from a joint. I asked him if he'd eaten any of the chocolates. He said no. "I just made myself a sandwich." My heart sank. When he pointed to the knife he used to make the sandwich, he confirmed my fear. Poor dear, who barely puff-puffs and always passes, sat glued to the couch in a full-on green out for hours, watching the original Italian *Swept Away*.

As a cook and edible maker, I'd failed him. A microscopic amount of distillate stuck to the knife, and while I usually swirl the sticky knife in the hot cream to melt it off, this time I skipped that step. The paring knife had barely a smear of distillate on the edge, but $\frac{1}{10}$ of a gram of 90 percent distillate contains 90 milligrams of THC; it takes only the tiniest amount to get stoned. When he used my dirty knife, it transferred the distillate to the cheese, and his toasted sandwich toasted him.

When I prepare raw chicken, I use a plastic cutting board designated for raw meat and fish. Using a non-porous cutting board to avoid bacteria growth and reserving it only for raw meat reduces the risk of food-borne illness. Cooking with weed requires the same type of consideration.

Since that incident, I make sure to thoroughly wash my dishes immediately after making infused food, label all my edibles with the potency and date, and tell anyone staying in my home to check the labels before they dig in. Getting high on purpose usually results in a good time, but nobody, even the most massive stoner, wants the out-of-control feeling of an accidental dose.

MAGICAL WHIP

MAKES 1¼ cups

TIME: 10 minutes

DOSE: 20 mg THC
per tablespoon

My having grown up in a family that ate peanut butter, banana, and mayonnaise sandwiches might explain why this condiment is a must-have for my stash of staples.

1 / In a small bowl, stir together the vinegar, lemon juice, mustard, sugar, and salt and set aside.

2 / In a medium bowl, use a handheld mixer on medium speed to beat the egg yolk for a few seconds. Continue mixing while slowly dripping about ¼ cup of the oil into the egg yolk—drip it as if from an eyedropper until the emulsion starts to build, until the mayo thickens and whitens.

3 / Pause to scrape down the sides of the bowl with a rubber spatula and add a splash of the vinegar mixture. Then continue blending and drizzling in another ¼ cup of the oil. Repeat with the third ¼ cup of oil. Continue beating and add the rest of the vinegar mixture, then the rest of the oil. Mix the mayo until it looks white, thick, and jiggly, then add the paprika and blend for another few seconds. Use immediately or keep in a labeled airtight container in the fridge for up to 2 weeks.

½ tablespoon white wine vinegar

½ tablespoon freshly squeezed lemon juice (about ½ a lemon)

1 teaspoon Dijon mustard

½ teaspoon granulated sugar

½ teaspoon kosher salt

1 large egg yolk

1 cup OOO Vegetable Oil (page 64)

Pinch of paprika

SERVING SUGGESTIONS:
The spread has a sweet tang that adds a zip to the Revved-Up Ranch (page 123) and can be spread on any sandwich for afternoon high tea.

ROASTED GARLIC COMPOUND CANNABUTTER

MAKES 1 cup

TIME: 1 hour 15 minutes

DOSE: 25 mg THC per tablespoon

My approach to edibles leans into the herbaceousness of the plant, and weed fits right into the classic compound butter, matching the herbs, spices, alliums, and other terpene-rich ingredients flavoring the fatty blank slate of butter.

1 / Preheat the oven to 400°F.

2 / Place the skin-on garlic cloves in the center of a piece of foil and drizzle with the olive oil. Wrap the foil around them, folding the edges together to enclose the garlic in a pouch. Place it in the center of the oven for 1 hour, then set aside to cool in the foil for 2 to 3 minutes before unwrapping.

3 / Squeeze the soft garlic cloves out of their skins and into a food processor. Add the cannabutter and purée until the garlic blends into small chunks and incorporates into the butter, 20 seconds. Use a rubber spatula to scoop the garlicky butter into a medium bowl and stir in the herbs, salt, and black pepper until the aromatics are evenly distributed, 30 seconds. Scoop the compound butter onto a piece of parchment paper and shape the butter into a rectangle using the paper and spatula. Fold the paper around the butter tightly and use a piece of tape to secure it. Alternatively, tablespoons of compound butter can be frozen on a parchment-lined sheet pan and then tossed into a freezer-safe bag. Just remember to label the dose.

8 large garlic cloves, separated, but with the skin still on

1 tablespoon olive oil

1 cup (8 ounces) Cannabutter (page 61), room temperature

¼ cup chopped soft fresh herbs (I like chives and parsley leaves)

1 teaspoon kosher salt

½ teaspoon freshly ground black pepper

SERVING SUGGESTIONS:
Melt this fragrant, garlicky butter into the filling of the Thrice-Baked Couch Potatoes (page 84), scoop it onto a juicy steak, or slather it onto crusty bread.

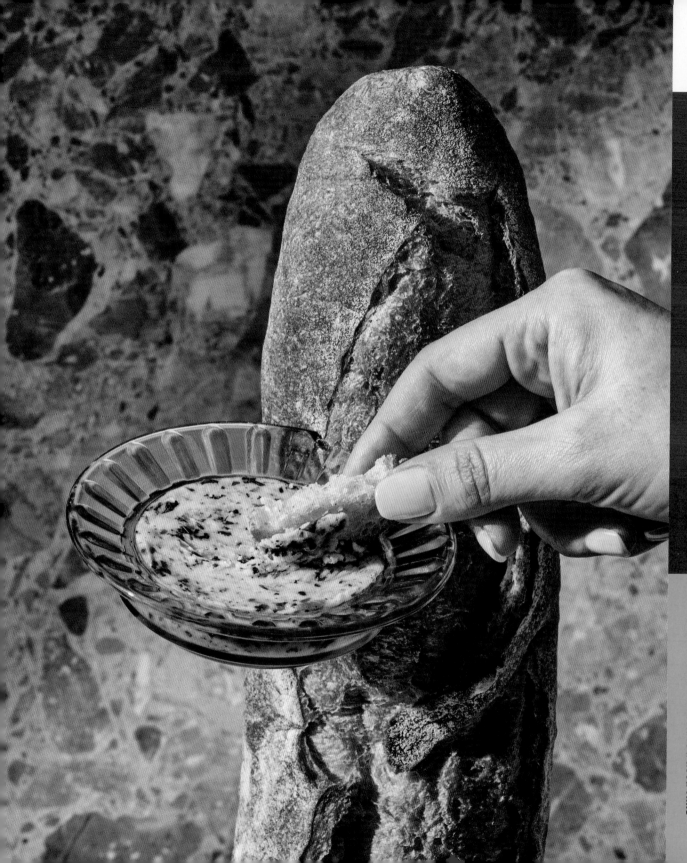

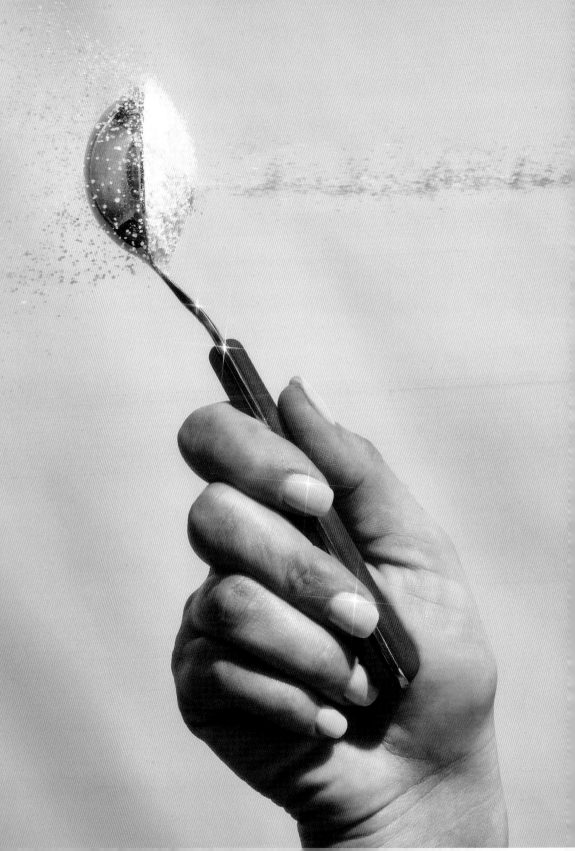

STONED SUGAR

MAKES 3 cups

TIME: 1 hour 20 minutes

DOSE: 10 mg THC per tablespoon

Mary Poppins knew a thing or two about a good time. Most of my mornings start with a spoonful of Stoned Sugar swirled into my tea to calm my nerves, and it kicks off my day in the most delightful way.

I use sugar more than any other ingredient in my pantry, and, when I want to infuse a recipe without using a liquid or oil, weed sugar steps up to the plate. As the alcohol in the tincture slowly evaporates in the oven, the sugar crystals get shellacked in the cannabis resin. Make sure the oven stays at a low temperature (a dehydrator works, too) so the sugar never melts but the liquid in the tincture evaporates.

1 / Preheat the oven (or dehydrator) to 180°F.

2 / In a medium bowl, use a rubber spatula to stir together the sugar and Turnt Tincture until the tincture is evenly distributed and the sugar looks like wet sand. Spread the wet sugar on a half sheet pan and bake for 75 to 90 minutes, stirring every 30 minutes. The sugar will go from looking wet and clumpy to a dry silt. If big chunks of sugar form, blitz the whole batch in a food processor for a few seconds. Store in a labeled airtight container for up to 3 months.

3 cups granulated sugar

½ cup Turnt Tincture (page 70)

The Pot Pantry

How to Eat Weed & Have a Good Time

WHIPPED WEED HONEY

MAKES ½ cup

TIME: 5 minutes

DOSE: 6.25 mg THC
per tablespoon

My aunty Yo started making infused weed honey and swirling it into her breakfast tea to replace her morning joint and soothe her throat. At first, she put the weed directly into the honey, but it had little effect: THC binds to fat and suspends in alcohol, but honey contains neither. Since the water content in a tincture would crystallize honey, the best way to dose it incorporates a little bit of fat—in this case, blending in OOO Coconut Oil (page 64). This process breaks up the crystals and whips the honey into an aerated, spreadable, spoonable cream, sweet enough to stir into smoothies, melt into a cup of tea, or slather on toast with a sprinkle of cinnamon.

In a stand mixer fitted with the paddle attachment, mix the honey and coconut oil on high speed until thick and lighter in color, and creamy, 4 to 5 minutes. Transfer to a labeled airtight container and store at room temperature, or in the fridge, where it will stay homogenized for up to a month.

6 tablespoons honey

2 tablespoons OOO Coconut Oil (page 64)

HEADS UP, POTHEAD!
Because this recipe blends any crystals out of the honey, it's a great way to use up an old jar in the back of your pantry.

POT PEANUT BUTTER

MAKES 2 cups

TIME: 45 minutes

DOSE: 12.5 mg THC
per ¼ cup

Americans eat enough peanut butter in a year to coat the floor of the Grand Canyon, making it essential enough to earn a place on the shelf of the pot pantry. Smearable nuts are an easy way to dose almost anything, like a pot-nut butter sandwich or ants high on a log. Americans also have strong feelings about their peanut butter texture, but, thankfully, this one works for everyone, so customize for your preference. The longer the peanut butter blends, the smoother it gets. Chunky lovers can also add extra finely chopped peanuts at the end.

1 / Preheat the oven to 240°F.

2 / In a large, oven-safe ramekin, bake the oil for 10 minutes, then check that the oil is 240°F before continuing. Use a small whisk to vigorously stir the flower into the heated oil. Leave it in the oven for 20 more minutes, stirring every 5 minutes, then pour the infused oil through a cheesecloth-lined strainer into a bowl. Let the flower cool for a few minutes, then gather the cheesecloth and squeeze out the last drops of infused oil. Save 2 tablespoons of this double-strength oil for a future project and use 2 tablespoons in the peanut butter.

3 / In a food processor, blend the peanuts, honey, salt, and 2 tablespoons of the infused oil until smooth, without any gritty chunks. It will take 8 to 10 minutes, but stop the machine and use a rubber spatula to scrape down and redistribute the peanut butter after 5 minutes. Store in a labeled airtight container in the fridge for up to 2 months.

¼ cup peanut oil

1 gram decarboxylated ground flower

3 cups unsalted roasted peanuts

3 tablespoons honey

1 teaspoon kosher salt

HEADS UP, POTHEAD!
This recipe makes ¼ cup of double-strength infused oil but uses only two tablespoons. Use the extra infused oil in the Cosmic Chili Crisp (page 124) or any other recipe that needs more potency.

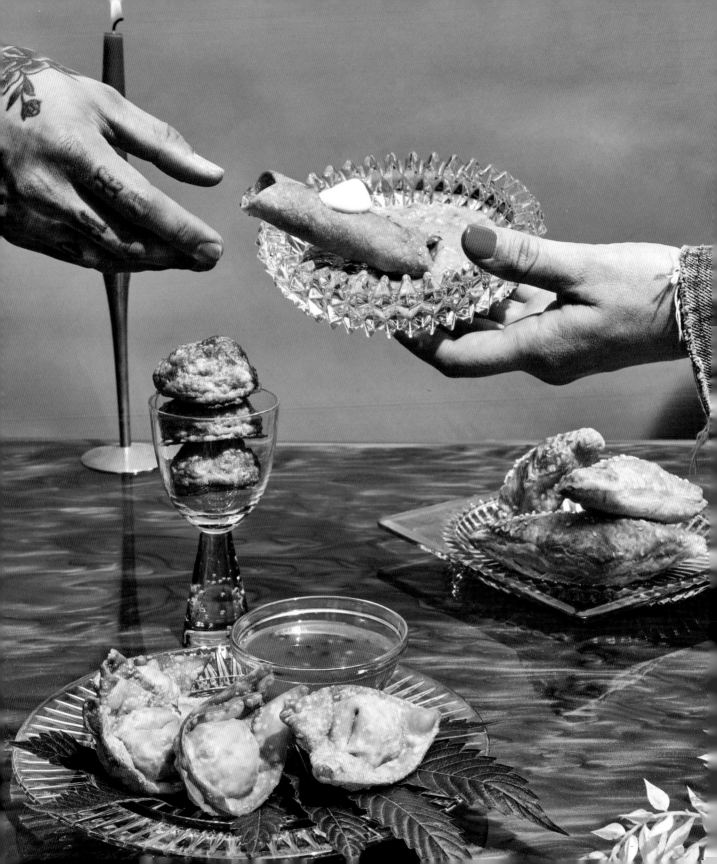

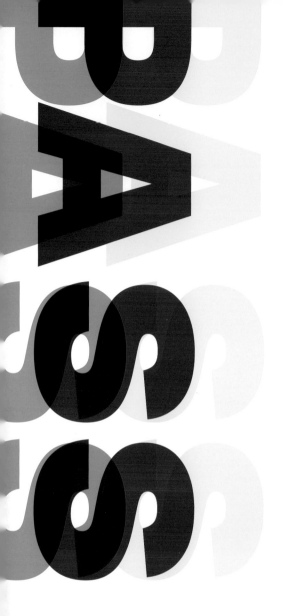

HIGHLY SHAREABLE SAVORY BITES

Bring the most talked-about app to the potluck, offer a platter of expertly dosed hors d'oeuvres at a high housewarming, or kick off cannabis karaoke night with infused nibbles. Whatever the occasion, these handheld snacks spark the conversation as you pass the dish on the left-hand side.

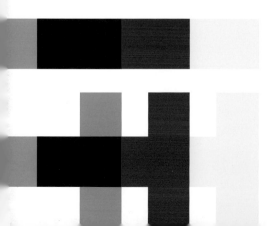

TOKER TAQUITOS

MAKES 34
taquitos

TIME: 1 hour

DOSE: 1.5 mg THC
per taquito

Taquitos are the smaller cousin of flautas, the fried friend of tacos, and a crispy, dippable finger food. They deliver the stoner trifecta of textures: crunchy, cheesy, creamy. In this vegetarian recipe, the corn tortilla tucks around the cumin-seasoned bean filling and rolls up tightly, just like a joint.

1 / In a 3-quart saucepan over medium-low heat, warm the olive oil for 1 minute, then add the onion and sprinkle with the salt. Cook the onion, stirring frequently, until translucent but stopping before it caramelizes, about 5 minutes. Add the garlic and cumin and stir for another minute. Add 1 tablespoon of adobo sauce from the can and stir until the sauce coats the onions and caramelizes, 1 to 2 minutes. Add the beans and water or stock, stir to mix everything together, then stir every minute for 5 more minutes. Remove from the heat and set aside.

2 / In a clean kitchen towel, wrap 10 tortillas and microwave for 30 seconds, so they become soft and pliable. Work with 1 tortilla at a time, keeping the rest tucked into the towel to stay warm. Place the tortilla on a plate and scoop 1 tablespoon of beans onto the bottom third of the tortilla. Use the back of the spoon to spread the beans flat. Sprinkle with 1 tablespoon of cheese.

3 / Roll the tortilla all the way up, like a joint, then place the taquito on a sheet pan with the seam facing down. Repeat with the remaining tortillas and beans.

4 / Place a wire cooling rack on a sheet pan and set it next to your frying station. Place a 10-inch sauté pan over medium heat for 1 minute, then add ¼ cup of oil and let it warm up for 4 minutes. Use tongs to set 5 or 6 taquitos at a time into the pan, seam-side down. Carefully rotate them as they cook, staying mindful of splattering hot oil. Cook until golden brown all over, 4 to 5 minutes. Transfer to the wire rack to cool and repeat with remaining taquitos. Halfway through frying, use the final ¼ cup of oil to replenish the pan, allowing it to heat up for 4 minutes before frying again.

5 / Top the taquitos with sour cream and shredded lettuce and serve immediately.

2 tablespoons OOO Olive Oil (page 64)

½ cup diced white onion (about ½ small onion)

½ teaspoon kosher salt

2 garlic cloves, minced

½ tablespoon ground cumin

1 (7-ounce) can chipotle peppers in adobo sauce

1 (16-ounce) can refried beans

2 tablespoons water or vegetable stock

34 (4-inch) corn tortillas (often labeled street taco)

2½ cups (10 ounces) grated pepper jack cheese

½ cup neutral oil such as vegetable or canola for frying, divided

Sour cream, for serving

Shredded iceberg lettuce, for serving

SERVING SUGGESTION:
Dunk them in the Ganja Guacamole (page 113) and Grass Is Greener Salsa Verde (page 112) to make it a fiesta.

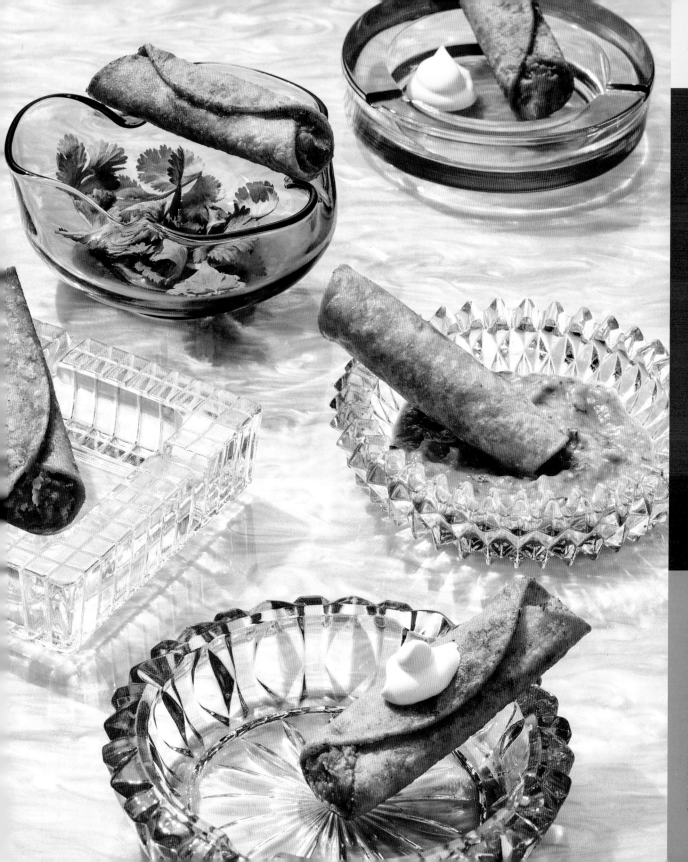

How to Eat Weed & Have a Good Time

THRICE-BAKED COUCH POTATOES

MAKES 24 servings

TIME: 2 hours 30 minutes

DOSE: 6.25 mg THC per potato (2 halves)

Thrice-baked potatoes get a soft center on the first bake, a crackly skin on the second, and get everyone else baked in return on the third. For ideal handheld appetizers, try to find the smallest, roundest Yukon gold potatoes.

1 / Preheat the oven to 400°F.

2 / Line a sheet pan with foil, lay the bacon out flat, and put it into the oven for 16 to 17 minutes, until most of the fat has rendered and the bacon crisps up. Transfer the bacon to a wire rack or plate lined with a paper towel to cool. Pour most of the excess bacon fat into a small bowl, leaving behind just a thin layer on the pan. Set the bowl of fat aside for later.

3 / Use a fork to poke holes all over the potatoes, then roll the potatoes in the grease left in the pan. Bake the potatoes for 1 hour, rotating halfway through so the skin cooks evenly. Leave the oven on when taking out the potatoes and let them cool on the pan until comfortable to handle, about 10 minutes. With a sharp knife, cut each potato in half lengthwise. Use a melon baller or small spoon to scoop out two-thirds of the inside, leaving a small layer of potato on the skin for structure, and replace on the pan, open-side up. Put the potato innards in a medium bowl and set aside.

4 / Using a pastry brush, coat the inside of each potato skin with the reserved bacon fat and sprinkle all the potatoes with ½ teaspoon of salt. Return to the oven for 10 minutes.

5 / Mash the potato innards (or push through a ricer), then add the remaining ½ teaspoon of salt and the Compound Cannabutter. Stir with a rubber spatula until well combined.

6 slices thick-cut bacon

12 small Yukon gold potatoes

1 teaspoon kosher salt, divided

3 tablespoons Roasted Garlic Compound Cannabutter (page 74)

½ cup (2 ounces) grated sharp cheddar cheese

½ cup sour cream

¼ cup chopped fresh chives

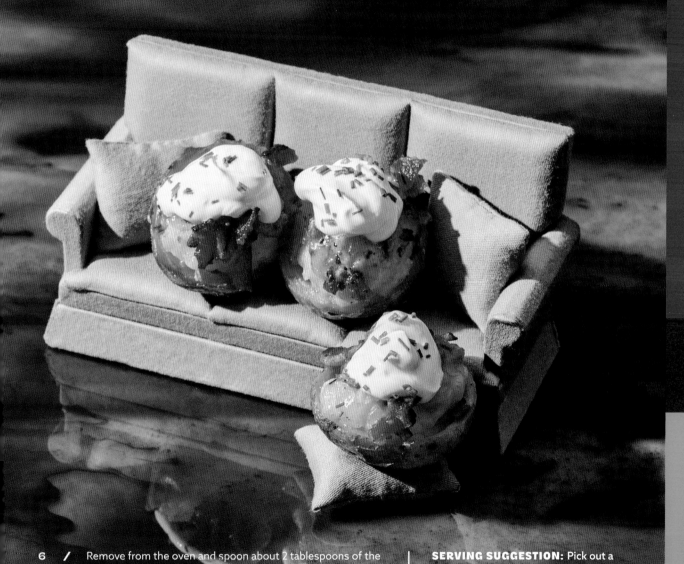

6 / Remove from the oven and spoon about 2 tablespoons of the dosed filling into each skin. In a small bowl, crumble up the cooked bacon and mix it with the cheddar cheese. Sprinkle the combination evenly over the tops of the potatoes and broil on high for 2 to 3 minutes, until the cheese gets bubbly and crispy. Let cool for a few minutes, then top with a small spoonful of sour cream and sprinkling of chives.

SERVING SUGGESTION: Pick out a show, call some friends, and whip up a batch of Bong Island Iced Tea (page 154) to ward off the cottonmouth.

CHICKEN POT POTPIES

MAKES 18 servings

TIME: 1 hour 20 minutes

DOSE: 5.5 mg THC per hand pie

With pot in the name, it only makes sense to add a little herb to the filling of these handheld chicken potpies. The buttery puff pastry, stuffed with a thyme-and-weed-seasoned chicken stew, bakes up into an impressive appetizer. Thankfully, these take only a stoner-level effort because they use frozen puff pastry and chicken from last night's rotisserie. Level up the laziness by freezing the handheld pies before baking: They stay good for up to six months in the freezer and impress at any impromptu rendezvous.

1 / In a 3-quart saucepan over medium heat, stir together the butter and oil until melted. Add the onion and cook, stirring, until it becomes slightly translucent, 5 to 6 minutes. Add the garlic, salt, flower, and paprika and keep stirring as everything sizzles in the fat for another minute. Add the flour and cook, stirring, for another minute, then pour in the chicken stock and heavy cream. Stir the pot, scraping the sides, until the liquid thickens and bubbles in the center for a minute. Turn off the heat and stir in the chicken, vegetables, thyme, and black pepper until the vegetables disperse throughout the filling and everything gets coated in gravy. Let the filling cool fully to room temperature before assembling, about 30 minutes.

2 / Preheat the oven to 400°F. Line two sheet pans with parchment paper.

3 / Dust a work surface with flour and lay out the puff pastry. Roll each sheet of puff pastry into a 10-inch square. Cut each square into 3 sections in both directions, making 9 squares from each sheet.

4 / In a small bowl, use a fork to beat together the egg and tablespoon of water. Dip a pastry brush in the egg wash and use it to wet the edges of a square, then place a heaping tablespoon of filling in the center. Fold the square diagonally, bringing the two opposite corners together to form a triangle. Pinch the triangle along the edges to seal the filling inside. Place the pie on the prepared sheet pan and press a fork along the edges, crimping and sealing the pastry. Repeat with the remaining squares of puff pastry. Use a paring knife to pierce

2 tablespoons (1 ounce) unsalted butter

1 tablespoon extra-virgin olive oil

½ cup finely diced yellow onion (about ¼ large onion)

2 garlic cloves, minced

2 teaspoons kosher salt

½ gram ground decarboxylated flower

¼ teaspoon hot paprika

3 tablespoons all-purpose flour, plus more for rolling

½ cup chicken stock

½ cup heavy whipping cream

1½ cups cooked and shredded chicken (about 1 breast)

1¼ cups frozen diced mixed vegetables

1 teaspoon minced fresh thyme

1 teaspoon freshly ground black pepper

2 (9.75 x 10-inch) sheets puff pastry, thawed

1 large egg

1 tablespoon water

Sesame seeds, for garnish

two small vents in the top of the pastry, then brush the tops of the pies with egg wash and sprinkle with sesame seeds. At this point, the finished, uncooked pies can be frozen for baking later.

5 / Bake for 18 to 20 minutes, until crispy and golden brown on top.

6 / Eat right away, when the pastry tastes best. Store in a labeled airtight container in the refrigerator for 2 to 3 days.

WACKY WEED WONTONS

MAKES 34 wontons

TIME: 1 hour

DOSE: 3 mg THC
per wonton

My aunty Yo and I have similar tastes in a lot of things, from gardening to weed, the latter especially when wrapped into these fried cream-cheese-stuffed wontons. Back in the day, she often ended up entertaining my uncle's surfer buddies, and as a vegetarian at the time, she adapted to what she had on hand in Kauai. These were always a big hit, and it helped that they freeze easily and she could fry them up later for a quick lunch or surprise guests. The Colman's mustard packs a punch of heat similar to wasabi, so Aunty Yo recommends offering guests soy sauce on the side to adjust the spice to their taste.

1 / In a small bowl, stir the mustard powder together with the water and let it sit for 10 minutes while you set up the mise en place for the wontons.

2 / In a medium bowl, use a rubber spatula or handheld mixer to blend the cream cheese, then stir in the celery, macadamia nuts, scallions, and flower.

3 / Add the soy sauce to the bowl of hydrated mustard and stir until fully blended, about 1 minute, then set aside.

4 / To assemble the wontons, scoop ½ tablespoon (about 6 grams) of the cream cheese mixture into the center of a wonton wrapper. Dip the tip of a pastry brush into the egg white and lightly brush the edges of the square wrapper. Fold the square in half diagonally, making a triangle, then push the air out from around the filling and pinch the edges together. With the wonton flat on the counter, the folded-over long edge facing you and tip of the triangle away from you, dab a little egg white on one of the other corners (not the tip). Bring those 2 corners together, overlapping and pressing firmly. The top triangle edge will flip up and create a shape similar to a hat. Set the wonton on a sheet pan lined with parchment paper to await frying.

2 teaspoons Colman's mustard powder

1 teaspoon water

1 cup (8 ounces) cream cheese

½ cup diced celery (about 1 stalk)

¼ cup roughly chopped macadamia nuts

2 tablespoons minced scallions (about 2 scallions)

½ gram ground decarboxylated flower

2 tablespoons soy sauce

34 square wonton skins

1 large egg white, whisked

6 cups neutral oil such as vegetable or canola for frying

Sweet chili sauce, such as Maggi, for serving

recipe continues

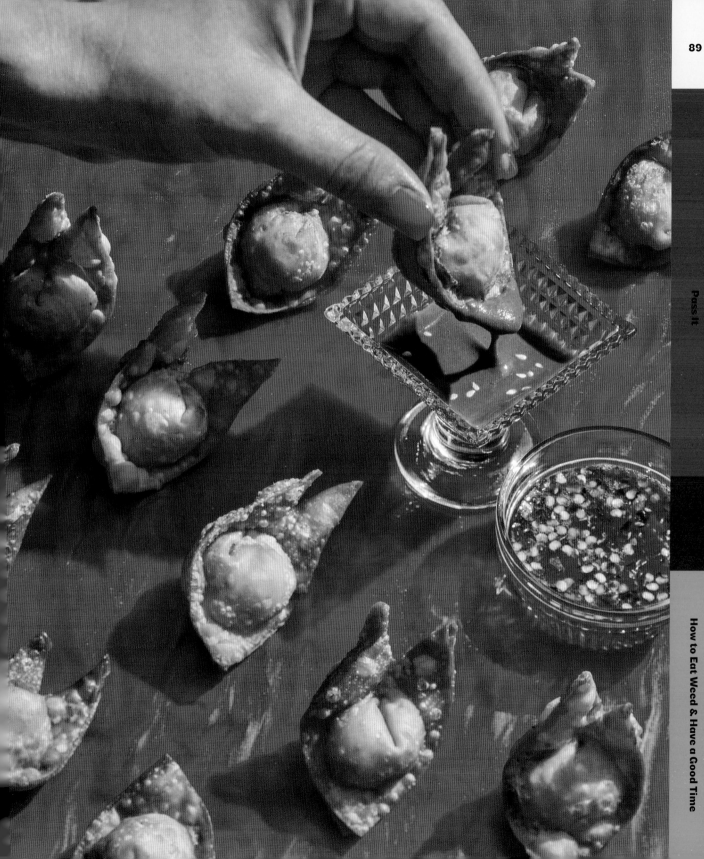

Repeat the process with the remaining wonton wrappers. For future cooking, label and freeze the wontons. To cook from frozen, add an additional 30 seconds to the frying time.

5 / In a heavy-bottomed pot or Dutch oven set over medium heat, pour the oil, making sure it fills more than half the pot but not more than two-thirds, to allow the oil to bubble up without spilling over. Bring the oil to 360°F, then adjust the heat as necessary to maintain the temperature while frying.

6 / Add the wontons to the oil 3 or 4 at a time, to avoid overcrowding the pot. Using a spider or large slotted spoon, flip the wontons after 2 minutes. Cook for another 2 minutes, until they turn crispy and golden brown. Use the spider to remove from the oil and place on a wire rack set over a sheet pan to cool. Repeat with the remaining wontons. Serve with the spicy mustard and sweet chili sauce.

HASH PUPPIES

MAKES 25 hash
puppies

TIME: 30 minutes

DOSE: 2 mg THC
per puppy

Be careful snacking on these cloudlike cornmeal fritters
while frying. The milligrams sneak up and frying while fried is
dangerous. When hash is on hand, swap out the cannabutter
for regular butter and add 10 milligrams of (50 percent)
decarboxylated hash. Hash, the unsung hero for cooking with
cannabis, reduces the grassiness while increasing the potency.
And then these puppies really live up to their name.

1   /   Prepare a sheet pan for the finished pups by lining it with
paper towels or arranging a wire rack over it. In a heavy-bottomed pot or
Dutch oven over medium heat, bring the oil to 350°F.

2   /   In a medium bowl, whisk together the melted cannabutter,
buttermilk, egg, honey, and salt. Add the cornmeal, flour, baking powder,
and onion powder and whisk again to completely combine. With a
rubber spatula, stir in the jalapeños, scraping down the sides of the bowl
and stirring until the pieces fully incorporate throughout the batter.

3   /   Use a tablespoon to scoop and gently plop 5 hash puppies at
a time into the hot oil, staying mindful of splashes. Aim to keep the oil
at 350°F as the puppies cook until golden brown, about 2 minutes. Use
a spider or a slotted spoon to remove from the oil and transfer to the
prepared sheet pan. Sprinkle the puppies with salt, repeat with the
remaining pups, and serve immediately.

6 cups neutral oil such as vegetable or canola
for frying

2 tablespoons (1 ounce) Cannabutter
(page 61), melted

1 cup buttermilk, room temperature

1 large egg, room temperature

1 tablespoon honey

1 teaspoon kosher salt, plus more for
sprinkling

1½ cups fine white cornmeal (fine yellow
cornmeal also works, it's just a little less
sweet)

½ cup all-purpose flour

1½ teaspoons baking powder

1 teaspoon onion powder

3 tablespoons finely diced deseeded fresh
jalapeño pepper (about 2 peppers)

SERVING SUGGESTION:
To get the party barking, dip these golden
fritters into Revved-Up Ranch (page 123)
or BBQROFL Sauce (page 119).

DEVIL'S LETTUCE CUPS

MAKES 10 lettuce cups

TIME: 20 minutes

DOSE: 2.5 mg THC per lettuce cup

Thou shalt eat thy greens: Take a trip away from the stoner sweets and munchie madness with this handheld salad that doubles down on the healthful benefits of weed. These vegetable-forward cups evoke a retro era of entertaining and will inspire guests, vegetarian and omnivore alike, to thank the green Goddess.

1 / In a medium bowl, toss together the carrot, cucumber, tomatoes, peanuts, and jalapeño. Sprinkle with the salt and pour on the vinegar, then give the bowl another toss. Drizzle on the olive oil, stir again, and set aside.

2 / Scoop 1½ tablespoons of hummus into a lettuce leaf and smear it evenly down the interior spine. Pinch a chunk of alfalfa sprouts off from the mass of intertwined squiggles and stretch them out along the hummus. Repeat with the remaining leaves.

3 / Stir the cucumber, tomato, and carrot salad one more time, then spoon 1 tablespoon on top of the sprouts on each leaf. Top with 1 slice of avocado and a generous pinch of cilantro. Eat immediately.

1 cup peeled and grated carrot (about 2 carrots)

1 cup small-diced cucumber (about 1 large cucumber)

1 cup halved cherry tomatoes

½ cup chopped roasted peanuts

1 fresh jalapeño pepper, seeded and minced

½ teaspoon kosher salt

1 tablespoon red wine vinegar

3 tablespoons extra-virgin olive oil

1 cup Hemp Hummus (page 122)

10 leaves romaine heart or butter lettuce

½ cup alfalfa sprouts

1 avocado, cut into 10 slices

1 bunch fresh cilantro, leaves only, for garnish

SERVING SUGGESTION:

To connect with a higher power, drizzle with the Cosmic Chili Crisp (page 124).

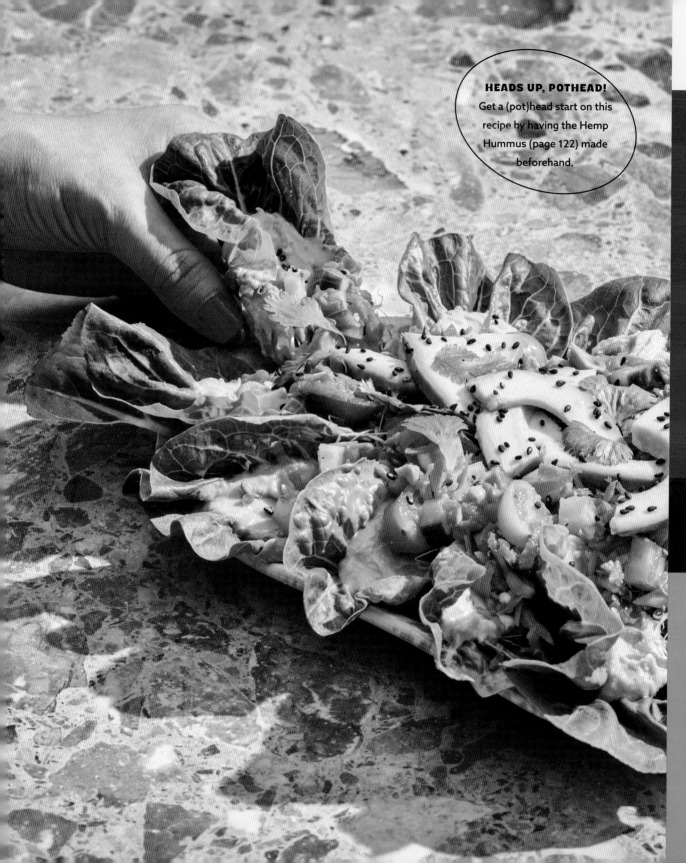

HEADS UP, POTHEAD!
Get a (pot)head start on this recipe by having the Hemp Hummus (page 122) made beforehand.

GREEN GOUGÈRES

MAKES 48
gougères

TIME: 1 hour 30
minutes

DOSE: 1 mg THC
per gougère

As a kid, my family called me Olive Oyl, as in Popeye the Sailor's lanky girlfriend who fed him spinach whenever he needed a boost of energy. I owned the nickname and ate a lot of spinach growing up, but my favorite way to eat my greens comes from my friend Alexander Roberts, a pastry chef. He baked a version of these cheesy green gougères for a dinner party and I adapted the recipe to include even more herb.

1   /   Center a rack in the oven and preheat the oven to 420°F.

2   /   Line two sheet pans with parchment paper.

3   /   In a blender, combine the water, milk, spinach, parsley, basil, and salt and blend on medium until puréed.

4   /   In a 3-quart saucepan over medium heat, combine the liquid greens with the butter and flower. Stir with a wooden spoon until the butter melts, then dump the flour in. Stir vigorously until it comes together as a dough, pulls away from the sides, and leaves a thin film on the bottom of the pot, 1 to 2 minutes. Transfer the dough to a medium bowl.

5   /   While the dough is still hot, use a handheld mixer on low speed to incorporate each egg into the batter before adding the next. The batter should look shiny and smooth, but not runny. If you pinch a bit of batter between two fingers, it should stretch at least an inch before breaking.

6   /   Blend in ¼ cup each of the two cheeses and then the black pepper, until evenly mixed throughout the batter. Using a tablespoon measure, scoop 24 cheese puffs per lined sheet pan, placing them 1½ inches apart. In a bowl, mix together the remaining ¾ cup of Parmesan cheese and ¼ cup of cheddar cheese. Sprinkle each puff with a pinch of the mixed cheeses.

7   /   Bake the first sheet pan for 25 to 30 minutes, until the bottoms turn a golden brown and the ridges of the tops get some color. Remove from the oven and bake the second sheet pan. Transfer to a wire rack, poke a small hole in the side of each gougère with a paring knife, and let cool for a few minutes before eating. The gougères freeze well in a labeled zip-top plastic bag. Re-crisp them on a parchment-paper-lined sheet pan in a 350°F oven for 22 to 24 minutes.

⅔ cup water

⅓ cup milk

2 cups (2 ounces) fresh baby spinach leaves

¼ cup fresh flat-leaf parsley leaves

¼ cup fresh basil leaves

½ teaspoon kosher salt

½ cup (8 ounces) unsalted butter

¼ gram ground decarboxylated flower

1 cup (120 grams) all-purpose flour

3 large eggs

1 cup (2 ounces) finely grated Parmesan cheese, divided

½ cup (2 ounces) grated sharp white cheddar cheese, divided

½ teaspoon freshly ground black pepper

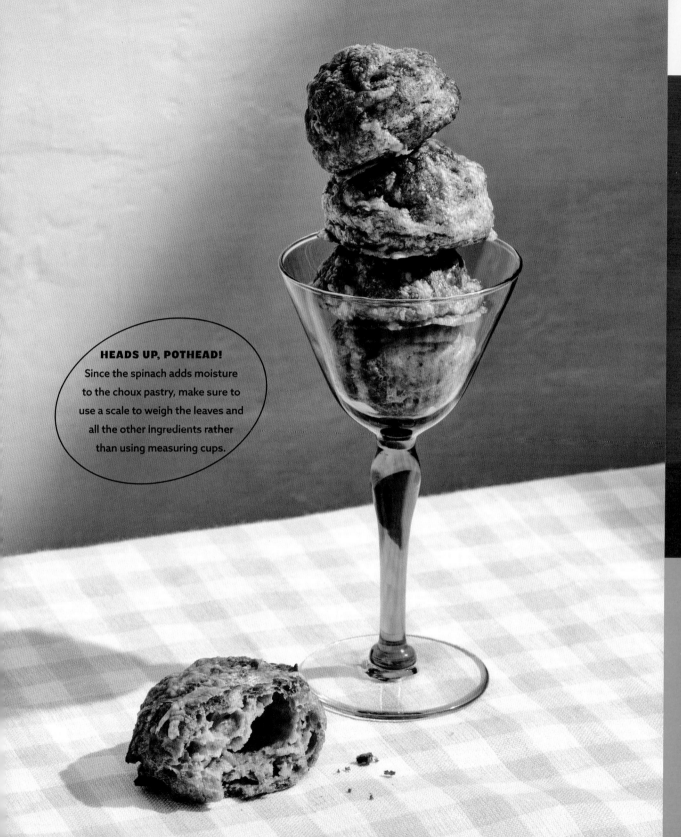

HEADS UP, POTHEAD!
Since the spinach adds moisture
to the choux pastry, make sure to
use a scale to weigh the leaves and
all the other ingredients rather
than using measuring cups.

HERBACEOUS MEATBALLS

MAKES 40 meatballs

TIME: 2 hours 30 minutes

DOSE 2.5 mg THC

Mint, the secret to my Sicilian grandma's meatballs, grows like a weed and (along with actual weed) gives these meatballs the extra herbaceousness that makes them special. Blending in lots of fresh mint complements any strain of pot, and the ricotta-soaked bread crumbs give these meatballs their irresistibly tender bite. Make these meatballs a day ahead and store them in their own sauce—they only get better as they marinate.

1 / In a small bowl, use a spoon to gently stir together the ricotta and bread crumbs. Set aside for 5 minutes to allow the bread crumbs to absorb the moisture from the ricotta.

2 / In a large bowl, use a rubber spatula (or your clean hands, as Grandma did) to mix the ricotta-soaked bread crumbs, pork, beef, Parmesan, mint, parsley, eggs, garlic, 1½ teaspoons of salt, pepper, and flower until thoroughly combined, but only just so. Divide the resulting mixture into 40 pieces (about 40 grams each), then form each piece into a meatball by slapping it back and forth between cupped palms a few times. My friend Frankie taught me this trick in Rome—it helps compact the balls and get the air bubbles out. Just 4 to 5 times should be plenty for the seams to disappear and the surface to look smooth—any more will overwork the ball. Roll the meat lightly between both palms to make it back into a round ball. Set on a sheet pan and repeat with the remaining pieces.

3 / Set a large heavy-bottomed sauté pan with a lid over medium heat for 2 minutes. Add the olive oil to the pan and lower the heat to medium-low for another 2 minutes, swirling the oil around the pan throughout. Working in batches, brown the meatballs in the pot, using tongs to rotate each meatball so that all the sides cook evenly. Continue to rotate the meatballs every 2 to 3 minutes for a total of 15 minutes to form an even brown crust all over. Place the cooked meatballs on the sheet pan (don't worry about doneness—they get cooked again) and cook the second half of the meatballs.

1 cup whole-milk ricotta

⅔ cup fine bread crumbs

1½ pounds ground pork

½ pound ground beef

1 cup (2 ounces) finely grated Parmesan cheese

⅔ cup chopped fresh mint leaves

⅔ cup chopped fresh parsley leaves

2 large eggs

8 garlic cloves, minced

3 teaspoons kosher salt, divided

1 teaspoon freshly ground black pepper

1 gram leftover Mota Milk flower (or ½ gram ground decarboxylated flower)

¼ cup extra-virgin olive oil

2 (28-ounce) cans peeled whole tomatoes

2 cups water

recipe continues

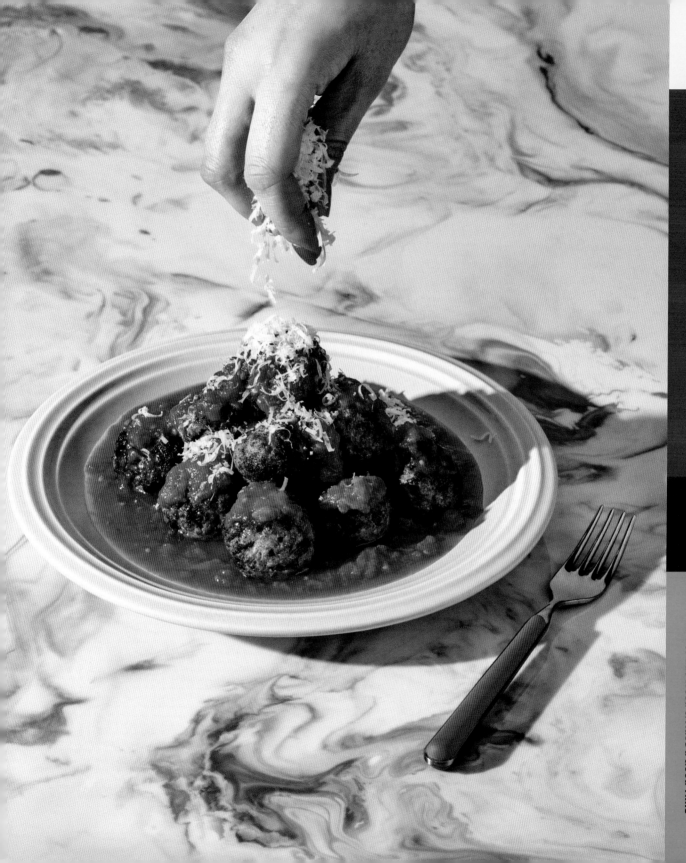

4 / While the meatballs cook, pour the tomatoes into a medium bowl, but save the cans. Use your hands to remove any hard tomato cores or stem nubbins and to squish the tomatoes to break them up. When the final batch of meatballs is cooked, add the rest back to the pan, add the tomatoes and remaining 1½ teaspoons of salt, and turn the heat down to low. Pour 1 cup of water into each of the tomato cans, slosh the water around, and add the liquid to the pan. With a wooden spoon or rubber spatula, give the meatballs a gentle stir, then cover, with the lid slightly cracked to let out steam. Cook for 1 hour on low heat, stirring every 15 to 20 minutes. Enjoy hot off the stove or wait—the meatballs taste even better the next day. Store the meatballs in a labeled, covered glass container for up to 5 days, then reheat in a large saucepan over low heat for 10 to 15 minutes. They also keep in the freezer for up to a month.

REEFER RICE BALLS

MAKES 25 rice balls

TIME: 2 hours 45 minutes, plus overnight for chilling

DOSE: 2 mg THC per rice ball

I only make risotto to eat arancini, or rice balls. The crunchy bread crumb exteriors hold together the creamy rice filling and a gooey mozzarella cheese center, creating the ultimate cheese pull. Conveniently, transforming rich, weed-infused risotto into crispy-crusted deep-fried globes allows people to track how much weed they eat by the ball, rather than the spoonful.

FOR THE RISOTTO

1 / In a 2-quart saucepan, bring the vegetable stock to a simmer over low heat. In a 10-inch sauté pan, heat the oil over medium-low heat until the oil shimmers, about 1 minute. Add the onion and sprinkle with the salt, then use a spoon or rubber spatula to cook, stirring, until it turns translucent, 3 to 5 minutes. Add the garlic and stir for an additional 30 seconds. Add the rice and cook, stirring to toast it, until it gives off a slight nutty aroma, about 2 more minutes.

2 / Use a ladle to add just enough stock to barely cover the rice. As the rice absorbs the flavorful stock, stir frequently and continue adding more stock every minute or two so the grains stay submerged in liquid, but just barely. After 20 minutes, add the peas and any remaining stock. Continue to cook, stirring, until the rice comes together with the starches and creates waves rather than splashing when stirred, another 10 minutes.

3 / Turn off the heat, add the cannabutter, Parmesan cheese, and black pepper, and stir until well mixed into the risotto. Pour the risotto onto a sheet pan and let cool to room temperature, then cover with plastic wrap and place in the fridge overnight to allow the starches to gel.

FOR THE RISOTTO

3 cups vegetable stock

2 tablespoons extra-virgin olive oil

½ cup finely diced yellow onion (about ½ onion)

½ teaspoon kosher salt

1 garlic clove, minced

½ cup carnaroli or arborio rice

½ cup frozen peas

2 tablespoons (1 ounce) Cannabutter (page 61)

½ cup (1 ounce) finely grated Parmesan cheese

¼ teaspoon freshly ground black pepper

recipe & ingredients continue

FOR THE RICE BALLS

4 / Remove the chilled risotto from the fridge and line a second sheet pan with parchment paper. Lightly wet the palm of one hand and place 1 tablespoon of risotto in the center. Drop a mozzarella cube in the middle of the risotto and use the fingertips of your free hand to smoosh the risotto around the cheese cube, making sure the cheese gets fully encased, then use both hands to gently shape into a round ball. Repeat, using the remaining risotto, for a total of 25 rice balls. Chill the formed balls in the fridge for 15 to 30 minutes.

5 / Line up three shallow medium bowls, with a sheet pan at the end. In the first bowl, combine the flour with a pinch of salt and ¼ teaspoon of black pepper. In the second bowl, whisk the eggs with a pinch of salt and ¼ teaspoon of black pepper. In the third bowl, use a fork or spoon to stir together the bread crumbs, Parmesan cheese, oregano, another pinch of salt, and the last ¼ teaspoon of black pepper.

6 / In a heavy-bottomed pot or Dutch oven, heat the oil over medium heat to 325°F.

7 / Use your left hand to roll a rice ball through the flour, then your right hand to roll it through the egg. Use your eggy right hand to pick up the ball and drop it in the bowl of bread crumbs. Switch back to the left (dry) hand to roll it in the bread crumbs. To keep the dry hand clean, start by sprinkling some bread crumbs over the ball and gently shaking the bowl to roll the ball around in the crumbs before finishing it up and placing it on the sheet pan. Repeat with the remaining balls.

8 / Set up a wire cooling rack on a sheet pan, then place 4 or 5 balls at a time in the oil, leaving room to move around. Rotate as they fry, cooking until they turn an even brown color, 2 to 3 minutes. Use a spider or slotted spoon to transfer to the wire rack and sprinkle with salt. Repeat with the remaining balls.

9 / Serve these warm for that satisfying cheese pull. They can be kept in the fridge for 2 days and reheated in the microwave, toaster oven, or air fryer but will lose a bit of their crunch. Alternatively, freeze in a labeled freezer-safe plastic bag after the breading step and store for up to 2 months. To fry from frozen, add 2 to 3 minutes to the cooking time so the cheese fully melts.

FOR THE RICE BALLS

½ cup (4 ounces) cubed low-moisture mozzarella cheese

½ cup (60 grams) all-purpose flour

1 teaspoon kosher salt, divided

¾ teaspoon freshly ground black pepper, divided

2 large eggs

½ cup (60 grams) fine bread crumbs

½ cup (1 ounce) finely grated Parmesan cheese

1 tablespoon dried oregano

6 cups neutral oil such as vegetable or canola for frying

SERVING SUGGESTION:

Dip these cheesy fried balls into the Oregano Marinara (page 118) and Mamma Mia, it's a party.

HEADS UP, POTHEAD!
Start this one the day before, as the risotto needs to chill overnight before it can be shaped into balls.

SKY-HIGH PIZZA PIE POPPERS

MAKES 33 poppers

TIME: 2 hours, plus 3 hours to overnight for resting

DOSE: 2.5 mg THC per 3 poppers

These crispy, chewy crowd-pleasers pay homage to Hot Pockets, right down to the tongue-blistering burns if you eat the mozzarella, tomato, and pepperoni–stuffed pizza balls too fast.

1 / In the bowl of a stand mixer, whisk together both flours, the granulated sugar, 1½ teaspoons salt, and the yeast. Use a rubber spatula to stir in the olive oil and lukewarm water. Using the dough hook attachment, mix on medium speed until the dough comes together and pulls away from the side of the bowl, about 5 minutes. Cover the bowl with a damp kitchen towel and let it rest for 15 minutes to hydrate the dough.

2 / Remove the towel and mix the dough on medium speed for 5 more minutes, using a rubber spatula to scrape down the sides of the bowl halfway through. Grease a large bowl with the extra-virgin olive oil, then scoop the dough into the bowl and re-cover with the damp towel. Let it rise at room temperature until doubled in size, 2 to 3 hours, or in the fridge overnight, which gives it a deep, yeasty flavor. If it rises in the fridge, take it out and let it come to room temperature for half an hour before continuing.

3 / In a small bowl, use a spoon to stir together the tomatoes, oregano, and ½ teaspoon of salt. Let the tomato mixture sit for 5 minutes, then strain and discard the liquid.

1½ cups (180 grams) all-purpose flour, plus more for dusting

1½ cups (180 grams) bread flour

1 tablespoon (12 grams) granulated sugar

2 teaspoons kosher salt, divided, plus more for sprinkling

1½ teaspoons active dry yeast

1 tablespoon OOO Olive Oil (page 64)

1 cup lukewarm water

1 teaspoon extra-virgin olive oil, for greasing the bowl

½ cup drained canned diced tomatoes

1 teaspoon dried oregano

½ cup (4 ounces) low-moisture mozzarella cheese, cut into ¼-inch cubes

15 slices pepperoni, quartered

6 cups neutral oil such as vegetable or canola for frying

recipe continues

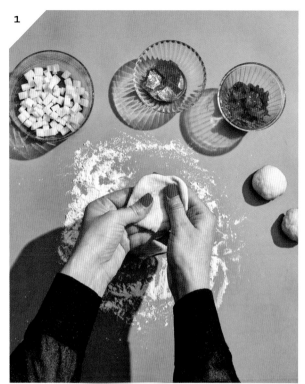

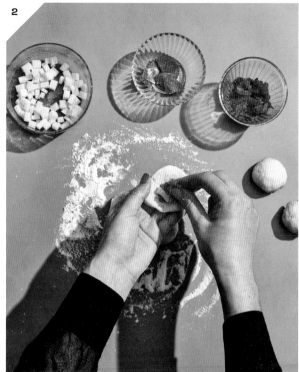

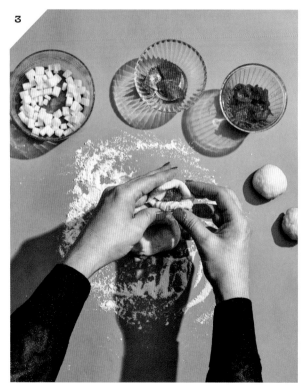

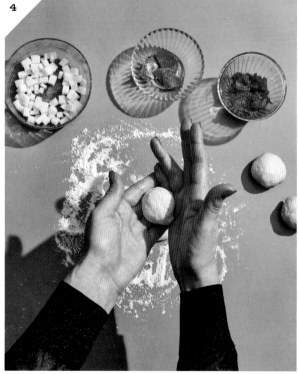

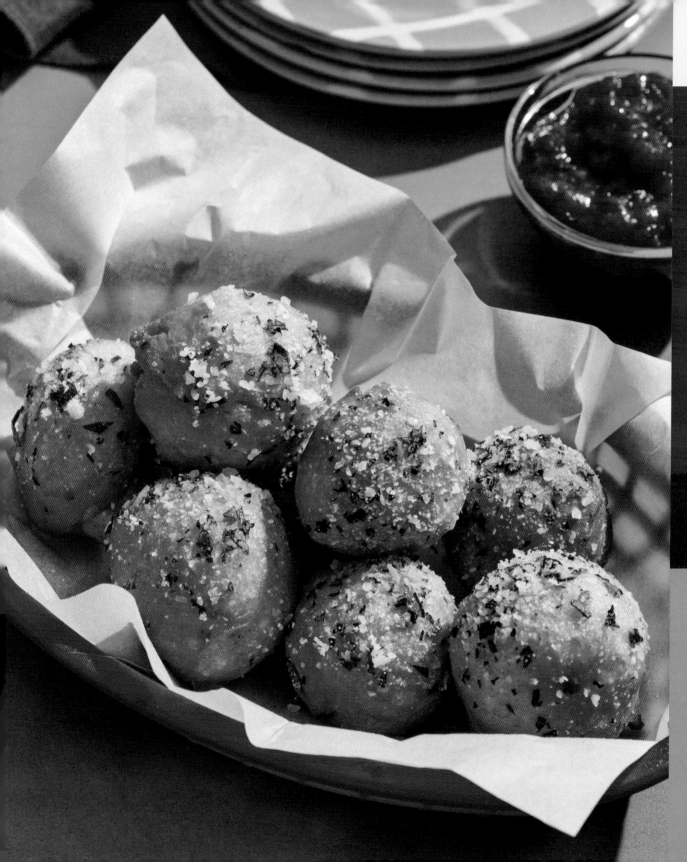

4 / Dust a sheet pan with flour and set it in a line with the bowl of salted tomatoes and 1 bowl each of cubed mozzarella and quartered pepperoni. Dust a work surface lightly with flour, then weigh out 33 even dough balls (about 16 grams each). Work with 11 balls at a time, keeping the remaining dough covered with a damp towel. Dust a small wooden rolling pin with flour and roll each ball into a 2½-inch diameter circle. In the center of each dough round, place 3 cubes of mozzarella, a chunk of seasoned tomato, and 2 pieces of pepperoni. Bring the edges of the dough together around the filling and pinch closed, like a purse, to seal the poppers. Place the finished poppers on the floured sheet pan and repeat with the remaining dough balls while the second person begins frying.

5 / In a large heavy-bottomed pot or Dutch oven, add the neutral oil, making sure it comes no more than two-thirds of the way up the side. Heat the oil on medium until it reaches 350°F, then aim to maintain that temperature.

6 / Line a sheet pan or plate with paper towels. Gently lower the poppers into the oil 3 or 4 at a time, stirring with a spider or slotted spoon to fry evenly. Cook until the outside turns deep golden brown, 4 to 5 minutes, then transfer to a sheet pan or plate and sprinkle with kosher salt. Repeat with the remaining poppers. Serve immediately; they taste best hot and fresh out of the fryer.

HEADS UP, POTHEAD!
Grab a classmate for this after-school favorite, as assembling these is a two-person job. One person stuffs, the other fries, and everything moves smoothly and quickly.

SERVING SUGGESTION:
If you're a frequent flier and want to take the party to a new altitude, add a side of Pot Pesto (page 114) or Oregano Marinara (page 118).

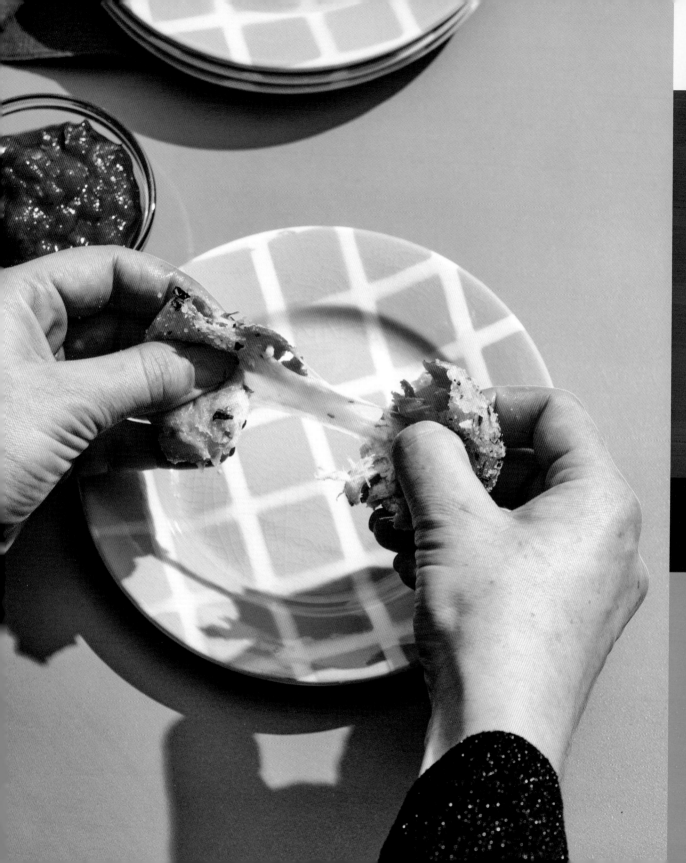

How to Eat Weed & Have a Good Time

STICKY ICKY POT-STICKERS

MAKES 24 pot stickers

TIME: 2 hours

DOSE: 2 mg THC per dumpling

I use store-bought wrappers for ease with these dosed dumplings, because I'd rather roll a joint than dough. The bottoms still brown up beautifully, cradling a juicy pork filling spiced with a pinch of Sichuan peppercorn and fresh ginger. The sweet twist of green apple balances the herbaceousness of the weed carried in the pork fat.

1 / In a food processor, blend the pork, cabbage, scallion whites, apple, soy sauce, ginger, fennel seed, Sichuan peppercorns, and flower until fully combined, 1 to 2 minutes. (You can also do this by hand in a large bowl.)

2 / Remove the dumpling skins from the packaging and set out a small bowl of water to act as the glue. Line a sheet pan with parchment paper for the finished pot-stickers. Measure the total weight of the pork filling and divide by 24. Weigh out 24 portions of filling equal to that amount (about 15 grams per dumpling).

3 / Scoop the measured filling onto the center of a dumpling skin. Dip your fingers in water, then dampen the rim of the top half of the dumpling skin. Fold into a half-moon shape, pinching only the center together. Pleat the front-facing right edge of the half-moon from the center toward the outer corner in a small fold and then gently pinch it together with the back edge of the wrapper. Repeat three or four times until the corner seals closed, then continue on the left edge of the dumpling. As you finish each dumpling, place it on the sheet pan. Continue until all the dumplings are filled and wrapped. Freeze the pot-stickers on the sheet pan until firm, 30 minutes. At this point, the finished, uncooked dumplings can be frozen for longer storage in a labeled freezer-safe bag for up to 3 months.

½ pound ground pork

½ cup minced green cabbage (about ⅛ head)

¼ cup minced scallion whites (about 4 scallions)

¼ cup peeled green apple, minced (about ½ an apple)

1 tablespoon soy sauce

½ tablespoon peeled and grated fresh ginger

¼ teaspoon ground fennel seed

¼ teaspoon ground Sichuan peppercorns

¼ gram ground decarboxylated flower

24 round dumpling or gyoza skins

6 tablespoons peanut or vegetable oil, divided

¾ cup water, divided

4   /   To cook the pot-stickers, place a medium sauté pan with a lid over medium heat for several minutes, then add 2 tablespoons of oil and heat for 1 to 2 more minutes. Cook 8 pot-stickers at a time, placing in the pan so each bottom sits flat, leaving about an inch of space between each dumpling, and fanning around the center of the pan. Turn the heat down to medium-low and fry until the bottom crisps and browns, 4 to 5 minutes. Add ¼ cup of water to the pan, which will spit. Quickly cover with the lid to steam. When all the water boils off, 5 to 6 minutes, remove the lid and turn the heat up to medium to crisp the bottoms of the pot-stickers, 2 to 3 minutes. Use a metal spatula to transfer the finished dumplings to a serving platter. Repeat the cooking process with each of the 2 remaining batches of the dumplings, using 2 tablespoons of oil and ¼ cup of water for each. Once finished, serve the dumplings immediately.

SERVING SUGGESTION:

I microdose these pot-stickers so everyone can have a few; to please the heavy hitters at the party, serve them with Cosmic Chili Crisp (page 124).

Pass It

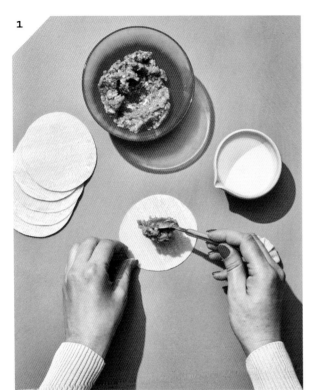

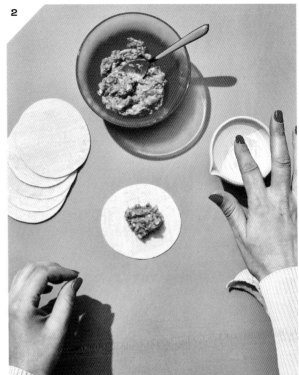

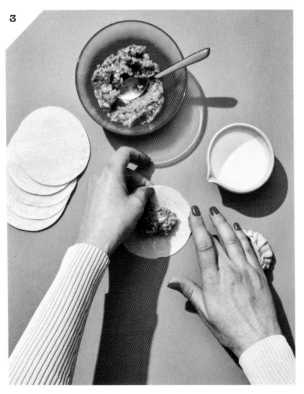

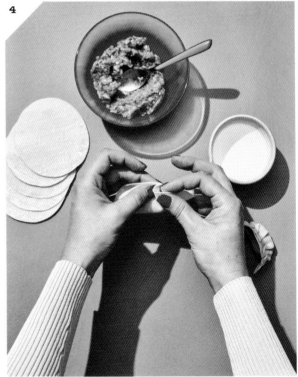

5

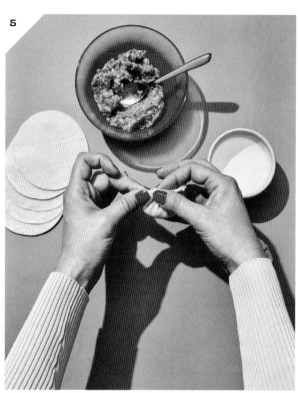

6

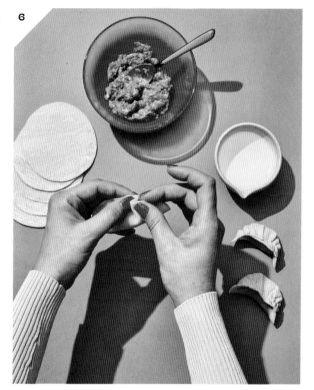

7

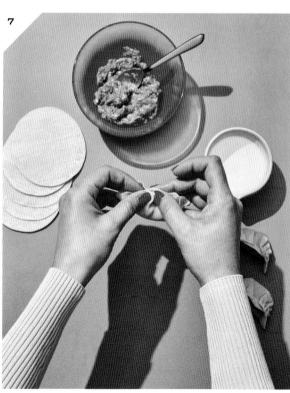

8

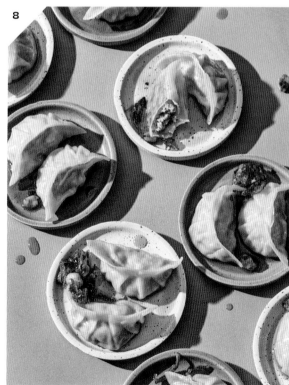

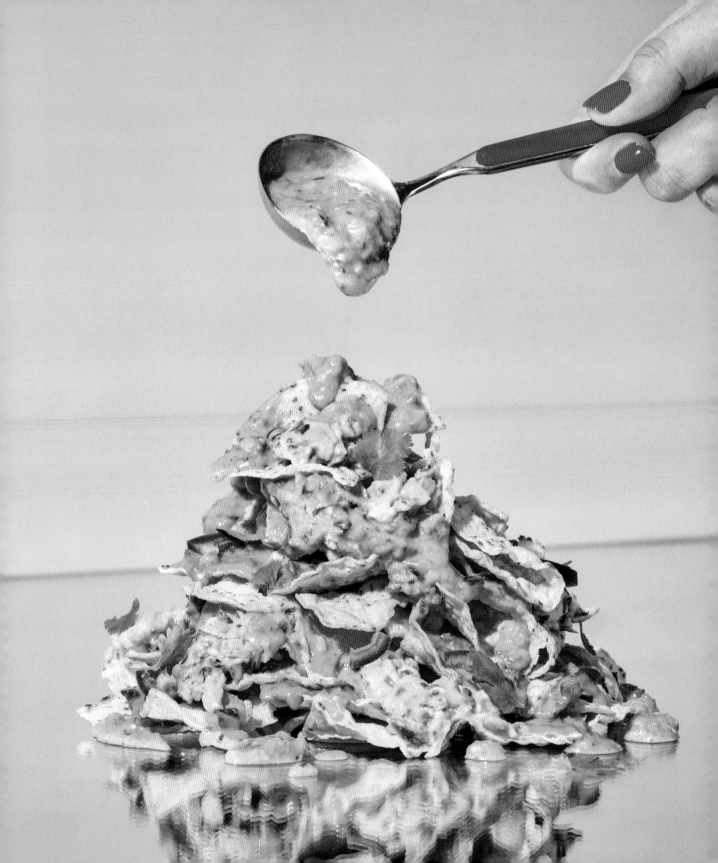

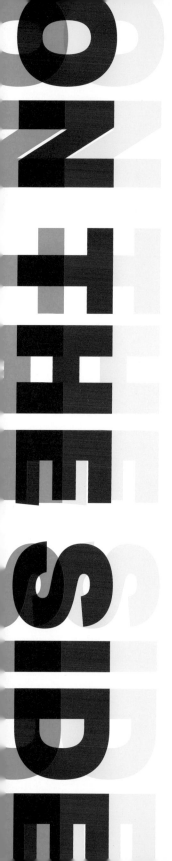

ON THE SIDE

INFUSED DIPS, DRESSINGS, AND SAUCES

A meal without a flavorful spread, zesty dressing, or crunchy accoutrement reminds me of an outfit without accessories. While Coco Chanel apocryphally said to remove one accessory, she was also a Nazi collaborator. I say put as many sides on the table as possible. As a bonus, keeping the mains mellow while dosing the dip allows guests to choose their own trip.

GRASS IS GREENER SALSA VERDE

MAKES 3 cups

TIME: 50 minutes

DOSE: 1 mg THC
per tablespoon

In the grocery store parking lot in LA's Echo Park, a metallic taco truck plastered with local band stickers blends up gallons of avocado salsa verde every day in anticipation of the late-night line of post-bar patrons. Having eaten a few gallons myself, and never grabbing enough tiny to-go salsas, I needed to make my own version of the creamy, spicy sauce, which incorporates a spoonful of weed-infused oil to take this salsa—and the party—to the other side.

1 / Preheat the oven to 420°F.

2 / On a sheet pan, spread the tomatillos, onion, garlic, jalapeño, and serrano and drizzle with the olive oil. Roast the vegetables for 30 to 35 minutes, until the tomatillos soften, get juicy, and their skins blister. The onion should take on a touch of color around their edges. Let cool for 10 minutes.

3 / Pour the vegetables, with their juices in the pan, into a food processor or blender and add the avocado, olive oil, and salt. Blend on low speed until the vegetables turn to a pulp, 1 to 2 minutes. Add the cilantro and lime juice and pulse 8 to 10 times, so the cilantro maintains just a semblance of a leaf. Taste and add more salt and/or acidity (with lime juice) to customize to your palate. Let the salsa cool completely before serving.

4 / Store any remaining salsa in a labeled airtight container in the refrigerator for 3 to 4 days.

1½ pounds tomatillos, husks removed, washed, and halved (about 12 medium tomatillos)

½ white onion, halved

3 garlic cloves, peeled

1 fresh jalapeño pepper, halved

1 fresh serrano pepper, halved

2 tablespoons olive oil

½ cup cubed avocado (about ½ large avocado)

2 tablespoons OOO Olive Oil (page 64)

1 teaspoon kosher salt, plus more to taste

½ cup chopped fresh cilantro leaves

¼ cup freshly squeezed lime juice (about 2 limes), plus more to taste

GANJA GUACAMOLE

MAKES 2 cups

TIME: 15 minutes

DOSE: 5 mg THC
per ½ cup

When I was growing up outside Edmonton, Alberta, avocados cost significantly more than they did in California, so my family used mayonnaise to stretch our guacamole and to give the dip a zing. Now I use a tablespoon of Magical Whip (page 73), because the egg in the mayo also helps homogenize the high—though a tablespoon of OOO Olive Oil or any other infused oil will work equally well.

1 / In a small bowl, pour ¼ cup of water over the diced onion to remove some of the pungency and set aside while preparing the other ingredients.

2 / In a large bowl, use a fork to lightly mash the avocado cubes and pour the lime juice over top. Stir in the cilantro, jalapeño, and serrano, then strain the onion and stir it in, too. Add the Magical Whip and salt, then stir until just mixed. Taste using the chips you plan to serve it with to check the flavor and add additional salt, if needed.

3 / Serve right away for the best-tasting guacamole. Store in a labeled airtight container, with plastic wrap pressed onto the surface, in the refrigerator for 1 to 2 days.

¼ cup water

¼ cup finely diced white onion
(about ½ a small onion)

3 avocados, cut into 1-inch cubes

¼ cup freshly squeezed lime juice
(about 2 limes)

½ cup minced fresh cilantro leaves and stems (about 1 bunch)

1 fresh jalapeño pepper, seeded and finely diced

½ fresh serrano pepper, seeded and finely diced

1 tablespoon Magical Whip (page 73)

1 teaspoon kosher salt, plus more to taste

SERVING SUGGESTION: Eat this guac with the Toker Taquitos (page 82) or some salty tortilla chips and salsa.

POT PESTO

MAKES 1 cup

TIME: 10 minutes

DOSE: 6.25 mg THC
per tablespoon

This recipe takes 10 minutes to make and stores wonderfully, putting a powerful pot of pot pasta within reach for quick weeknight dinners or lazy Sunday lunches. While it works atop roasted vegetables or slathered on toast, the real alchemy of this creamy Italian herb sauce comes when it fulfills its true destiny, as a pasta sauce. Since pesto concentrates the flavors of basil, combining just a tablespoon of pot pesto with a few tablespoons of the starchy water left after cooking your noodles creates a loose, silky sauce that coats every pasta shape.

1 / In a small sauté pan, toast the pine nuts on medium-low heat while swirling the pan until lightly golden brown, 3 to 4 minutes.

2 / In a food processor, purée the toasted pine nuts, garlic, and salt until they form a smooth paste (alternatively, this can be done with a mortar and pestle). Add the basil and purée while slowly drizzling in both olive oils. Add the Parmesan cheese and pulse a few times, just to mix. Store in a labeled airtight container in the fridge for up to a week or freeze for up to a month.

¼ **cup pine nuts**

3 garlic cloves

¼ **teaspoon kosher salt**

4 packed cups fresh basil leaves

¼ **cup extra-virgin olive oil**

¼ **cup OOO Olive Oil (page 64)**

1 cup (2 ounces) finely grated Parmesan cheese

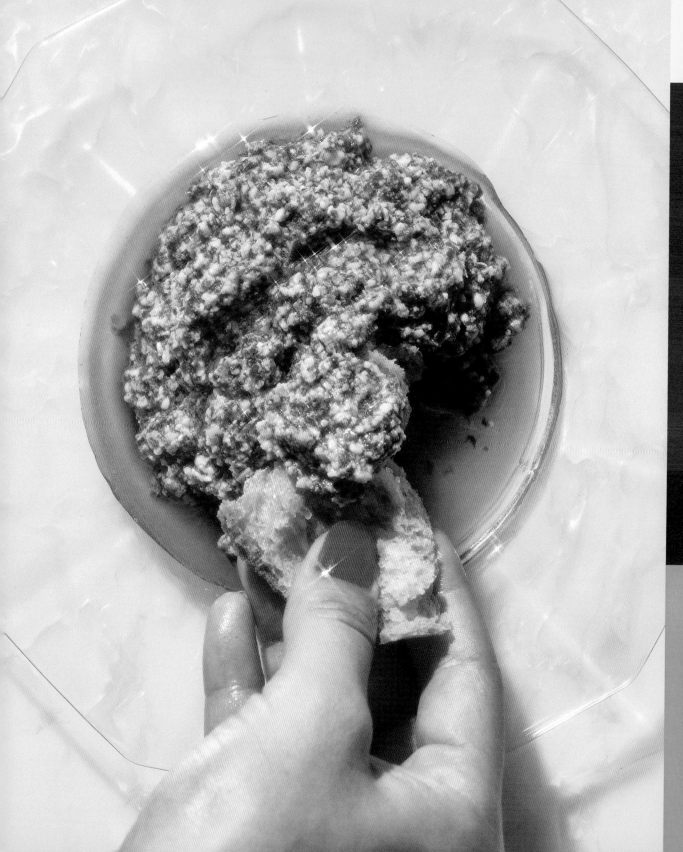

PETER PIPER'S PEPERONATA

MAKES 3½ cups

TIME: 1 hour 15 minutes

DOSE: 7 mg THC per ¼ cup

A Calabrian chef missing half a finger taught me how to make peperonata. While he never shared the story behind his pinkie stub, he did share his peperonata recipe (or, more accurately, technique). To almost confit the garlic and onion in the olive oil, he layered them on the bottom of the pan, then piled the sliced peppers on top, which steamed the onions below.

1 / Preheat the oven broiler.

2 / Cut the bell peppers into quarters and remove the stems, seeds, and white spines. Place the pepper quarters skin-side up on a sheet pan and broil, moving the tray around as necessary for even cooking, until the skin blisters and turns black, about 15 minutes. Remove from the oven and transfer to a lidded pot. Leave for 5 minutes; they will steam, making the skin easier to peel off. Peel the skins off of the peppers and cut into inch-wide slices.

3 / In a 3-quart saucepan with a lid, add the garlic, then layer the sliced onion on top. Sprinkle with ½ teaspoon of salt and pour both oils over top. Layer the pepper slices on top of the onion, sprinkle with the remaining ½ teaspoon of salt, and cover. Cook over low heat, undisturbed, for about 15 minutes. The layering of the ingredients creates steam and stews the garlic and onion in the olive oil. Remove the lid, letting the steam drip back into the pot, and add the tomato paste. Stir everything together, then replace the lid and cook for another 15 minutes, stirring every 5 minutes. Turn off the heat and stir in the red wine vinegar. Serve immediately or let cool to room temperature, pour into a labeled airtight container, and store in the fridge for 2 to 3 days.

6 red, orange, and/or yellow bell peppers

3 garlic cloves, peeled and smashed

½ medium yellow onion, thinly sliced

1 teaspoon kosher salt, divided

¼ cup OOO Olive Oil (page 64)

2 tablespoons extra-virgin olive oil

1 tablespoon tomato paste

1 tablespoon red wine vinegar

SERVING SUGGESTION:
Use peperonata to add a little edge to the Devil's Lettuce Cups (page 92), purée it into a creamy, vegetarian pasta sauce, or serve over toasted bread, like bruschetta.

OREGANO MARINARA

MAKES 6 cups

TIME: 1 hour

DOSE: 8.25 mg THC
per ½ cup

Growing up in an Italian American family meant we always had a pot of sauce bubbling away on the stove—or at least an old yogurt container full of it in the fridge. But my marinara evolved over the years, refining my bold, American, "more is better" attitude toward garlic. While cooking under a Calabrian chef in Rome, I learned an Italian technique that calls for removing the garlic from the sauce, leaving just subtle traces. Now, I take a middle-of-the-road strategy: Two smashed cloves flavor the oil, but only one stays in the finished sauce.

1 / In a heavy-bottom Dutch oven, heat the oil on medium-low for 1 minute. Add the smashed garlic, turn the heat down to low, and stir with a wooden spoon until the garlic turns golden brown, 1 minute. Transfer the garlic to a small bowl and set it aside.

2 / Sprinkle the flower and chili flakes into the pot, then pour in the tomato purée and stir, scraping the bottom and sides. Refill each of the empty tomato purée cans with 1 cup of the water to pick up the remaining purée. Add the cans of tomato water and the salt to the pot. Mince one of the reserved cloves of garlic to a paste, add it to the sauce, and stir well.

3 / Keep the heat on low and let the sauce cook, uncovered, stirring and scraping the sides with the wooden spoon every 5 minutes, until the sauce thickens and darkens to a brick red, an additional 45 minutes. Remove from the heat and stir the basil into the still-hot sauce. Let cool completely before storing in a labeled airtight container in the fridge for up to a week, or in the freezer for up to a month.

¼ cup extra-virgin olive oil

2 garlic cloves, smashed

½ gram ground decarboxylated flower

Pinch red chili flakes

2 (28-ounce) cans tomato purée

2 cups water

2 teaspoons kosher salt

1 bunch fresh basil, leaves only

SERVING SUGGESTION:
Put a bowl of this specially spiced sauce next to the Reefer Rice Balls (page 99), and *bong appetito.*

BBQROFL SAUCE

MAKES 2½ cups

TIME: 40 minutes

DOSE: 5 mg THC
per ¼ cup

Pitmaster Kevin Bludso kept his BBQ sauce spice blend top secret when we grilled together on *Bong Appétit*. But when we added weed into the mix, we shared a realization: Infused BBQ sauce hides the weed flavor and keeps the party lit. He never gave up the special mix for his BBQ sauce, but this tangy, spicy version brings flavor and entertainment to the event.

1 / In a 2- or 3-quart saucepan over medium-low heat, warm both olive oils and the garlic, stirring, until the garlic starts to smell fragrant, but doesn't take on any color, about 1 minute. Add the chili powder, cumin, sweet paprika, and cayenne pepper to the pan and cook, stirring, for 1 minute. Add the ketchup and cook, stirring to thicken, for 3 minutes.

2 / Add the beef stock, vinegar, molasses, and salt and stir to combine. Turn the heat to low and simmer, stirring every 5 minutes, until the sauce turns a rich mahogany color, about 30 more minutes. It should coat the back of a spoon and, if you run a finger through that coat, leave a clean streak. Take the saucepan off the heat and pour the sauce into a serving bowl or container to cool.

3 / Store in a labeled airtight container in the fridge for 2 weeks.

2 tablespoons OOO Olive Oil (page 64)

2 tablespoons extra-virgin olive oil

4 garlic cloves, minced

2 tablespoons chili powder

1 tablespoon ground cumin

1 tablespoon sweet paprika

1 teaspoon ground cayenne pepper

2 cups ketchup

½ cup beef stock (use vegetable stock or beer for a vegetarian version)

¼ cup apple cider vinegar

1 tablespoon blackstrap molasses

1 tablespoon kosher salt

SERVING SUGGESTION:
Dish this out as a dip, side-by-side with the Revved-Up Ranch (page 123), or spoon some on top of the Thrice-Baked Couch Potatoes (page 84).

On the Side

How to Eat Weed & Have a Good Time

QUESO EXTRA FUNDIDO

SERVES 8 to 10

TIME: 30 minutes

DOSE: 5 mg THC
per ¼ cup

Add too much weed to the queso and the fun-dido ends, as I learned throwing a party a few years ago. Now I dose the queso with the assumption that my guests will clean the skillet—nobody shows restraint in the face of ooey-gooey cheese. With all the mix-ins, this cheese dip stands up to the flavor of full flower or hash rather than an oil infusion. Plus, the cilantro, chili, smoky poblano peppers, and spicy chorizo work well with the flavors of weed.

1 / Heat a cast-iron skillet or large sauté pan over medium-low for 3 minutes. Add the olive oil to the pan and swirl it around, heating for another minute, then add the chorizo. Turn the heat to medium and use a spatula to break the pork into smaller pieces, cooking until the meat takes on a little bit of color and releases a bit of fat, but stopping before all the liquid cooks out, about 5 minutes. Use a slotted spoon to remove the chorizo from the pan and set aside in a bowl.

2 / In the same pan, add the scallion whites, garlic, and flower and cook, stirring, for a minute. Add the poblano peppers and continue to cook, stirring, until the peppers are tender, 6 to 8 minutes.

3 / In a small bowl, whisk together the cornstarch and tequila to make a slurry.

4 / In a small saucepan over low heat, warm the milks. Whisk in the slurry and raise the heat to medium until it boils, 2 to 3 minutes. Turn off the heat and stir in both grated cheeses, the cooked chorizo, jalapeño, poblanos, and ¼ cup of the cilantro. Use a rubber spatula to mix thoroughly until all the cheese melts and the ingredients are evenly distributed. Pour into a festive bowl and top with the remaining ¼ cup chopped cilantro and the scallion greens. Serve with chips and enjoy the dip while hot.

> **SERVING SUGGESTION:** Enjoy the dip on its own or atop nachos, layer it into a bean dip, or use it to load up a baked potato. For an extra dose, serve it with the Ganja Guacamole (page 113).

1 tablespoon extra-virgin olive oil

½ pound Mexican-style chorizo sausage, casings removed

2 scallions, whites and greens separated and minced

1 garlic clove, minced

¼ gram of ground decarboxylated flower

1 cup ¼-inch pieces of chopped fresh poblano pepper (2 large peppers)

1 tablespoon cornstarch

1 tablespoon tequila

1 (12-ounce) can evaporated milk

1 cup whole milk

1 cup (4 ounces) grated low-moisture mozzarella cheese

2 cups (8 ounces) grated Monterey Jack cheese

1 fresh jalapeño pepper, seeded and minced

½ cup chopped fresh cilantro leaves and stems, divided

1¼ teaspoons kosher salt

Tortilla chips, for serving

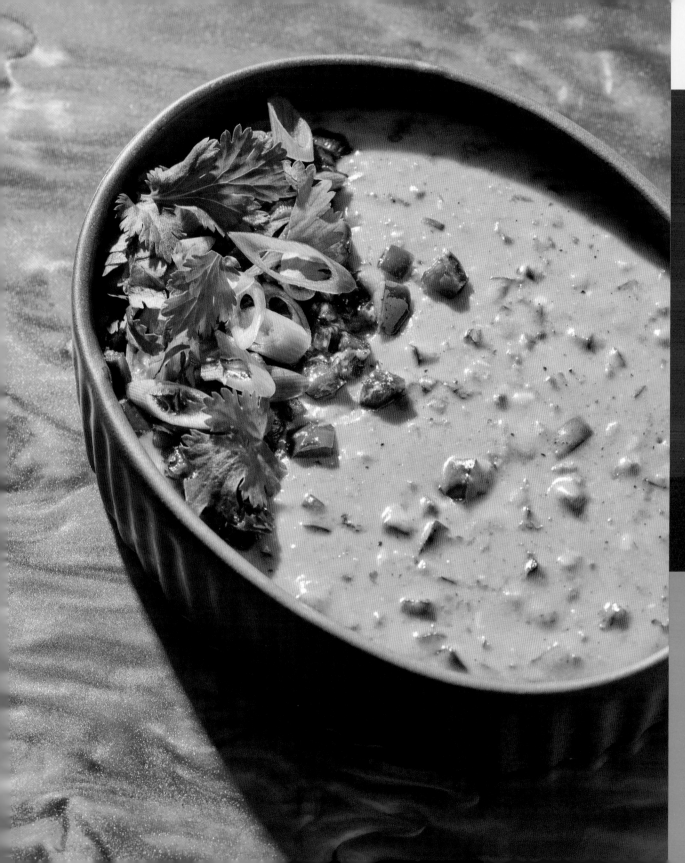

HEMP HUMMUS

MAKES 2 cups

TIME: 45 minutes

DOSE: 6.25 mg THC
per ¼ cup

When I asked an Israeli friend who makes the creamiest hummus I've ever tasted about using canned chickpeas instead of dried, he gave me the same look Italians give at the suggestion of cheese on fish. But damn, I love a tuna melt—and this weed-infused hummus made with canned chickpeas. If you enjoy the self-flagellation of soaking dried beans overnight and cooking them for many, many more hours than you even think possible, then go ahead and make hummus from dried beans. I would rather save the time and smoke more weed. Whatever route you take, the true secret to getting that restaurant-quality hummus lives in the skins. Or, rather, in their removal.

1 / In a 2-quart saucepan over low heat, combine the chickpeas, water, and garlic. Simmer, stirring occasionally, for about 20 minutes. Most of the skins will fall off the chickpeas and rise to the top. Skim off the skins from the top.

2 / Remove from the heat and use a slotted spoon to scoop the chickpeas and garlic into a food processor. Save the cooking liquid in case you need it to thin the hummus. Purée on high until it becomes smooth and fluffy, 2 minutes. Scrape down the sides of the bowl, then add both olive oils, the tahini, lemon juice, and salt. Purée for 2 more minutes, scraping down the sides halfway through. If the mixture is too thick, use the leftover cooking liquid to thin it to your preferred texture. Taste the hummus and adjust the seasoning as desired.

3 / Scoop the hummus into a serving bowl and use the back of a spoon to create peaks and valleys. Sprinkle with the smoked paprika, drizzle with olive oil, and nosh. To save the hummus for later, store in a labeled lidded container in the fridge for 3 to 4 days.

1 (16-ounce) can chickpeas, drained and rinsed

1½ cups water

3 garlic cloves, peeled

⅓ cup extra-virgin olive oil, plus more for finishing

2 tablespoons OOO Olive Oil (page 64)

⅓ cup tahini

¼ cup freshly squeezed lemon juice (about 2 lemons)

½ teaspoon kosher salt, plus more as preferred

⅛ teaspoon ground smoked paprika, for topping

SERVING SUGGESTION: Use this super-smooth hummus in the Devil's Lettuce Cups (page 92) or pack it with crudités to bring on a high hike.

REVVED-UP RANCH

MAKES 1½ cups

TIME: 10 minutes

DOSE: 3.25 mg THC
per tablespoon

Of all the dips in the world, ranch ranks number one in my book, thanks to its versatility: It makes raw broccoli taste good, cuts the heat of a spicy chicken wing, and goes fantastically on pizza (fight me!). This multifaceted condiment gets a tang from the buttermilk, and a bunch of grassy herbs give it color and flavor. Use whatever is available for those herbs: I often swap the dill for mint or the chives for scallions; sometimes I add marjoram. Blend up whatever looks tender and smells fragrant; as noted above, it's tough to go wrong with ranch.

In a food processor, pulse the mayonnaise, Magical Whip, sour cream, buttermilk, chives, parsley, and dill until the herbs look like specks and the dressing takes on a hint of green color, 1 to 2 minutes. Add the garlic powder, onion powder, Worcestershire sauce, pepper, and salt and pulse a few more times. Taste for seasoning, adding more salt or pepper to your preference. Pour into a serving bowl or into a labeled airtight container, which will keep it usable for up to 2 weeks in the fridge.

½ cup mayonnaise

¼ cup Magical Whip (page 73)

¼ cup sour cream

¼ cup buttermilk

¼ cup fresh chives

¼ cup minced fresh parsley leaves

¼ cup minced fresh dill

1¼ teaspoons garlic powder

1½ teaspoons onion powder

1 teaspoon Worcestershire sauce

1 teaspoon freshly ground black pepper

1 teaspoon kosher salt

COSMIC CHILI CRISP

MAKES 1½ cups

TIME: 30 minutes

DOSE: 4 mg THC
per tablespoon

My introduction to mala, the combination of the mouth-numbing spice of Szechuan peppercorns and the lingering heat of chilis, took place at a little Taiwanese spot on the outskirts of San Francisco's Inner Richmond called Spices II. The explosive chili flavor of their fried tofu converted me into a lifelong spice simp. This aromatic chili crisp captures that tingling heat—and a little extra twinkle—at home.

1 / In a heat-safe medium bowl, combine the Szechuan peppercorns, chili flakes, ginger, hot paprika, soy sauce, sugar, and peanuts, and set aside.

2 / In a 3-quart saucepan, heat the peanut oil on medium-low for 30 seconds, then add the shallots, garlic, flower, star anise, and cinnamon. Stir until the garlic and shallots begin to crisp and turn golden, 10 minutes. Turn the heat down to low and cook, stirring, until the garlic and shallots get fully crispy, an additional 8 to 10 minutes. The liquid in the garlic and shallots will prevent the oil from getting too hot and degrading the flower. Remove from the heat and use tongs to remove the cinnamon stick and star anise from the oil. Right away, pour the flavored oil over the bowl of spices and use a spoon to stir it all together, distributing the oil.

3 / Spice up your life immediately or keep the sauce refrigerated in a labeled lidded container for up to 3 months; it only gets tastier with time.

½ tablespoon Szechuan peppercorns, coarsely ground

¼ cup red chili flakes

2-inch piece fresh ginger, peeled and thinly julienned

1 tablespoon hot paprika

1 tablespoon soy sauce

2 teaspoons granulated sugar

¼ cup roasted salted peanuts

1 cup peanut oil

2 shallots, thinly sliced

12 garlic cloves, thinly sliced

½ gram ground decarboxylated flower

2 whole star anise

1 cinnamon stick

SERVING SUGGESTION:
Drizzle this crunchy, spicy, lightly dosed condiment on the Devil's Lettuce Cups (page 92) to reach a higher power.

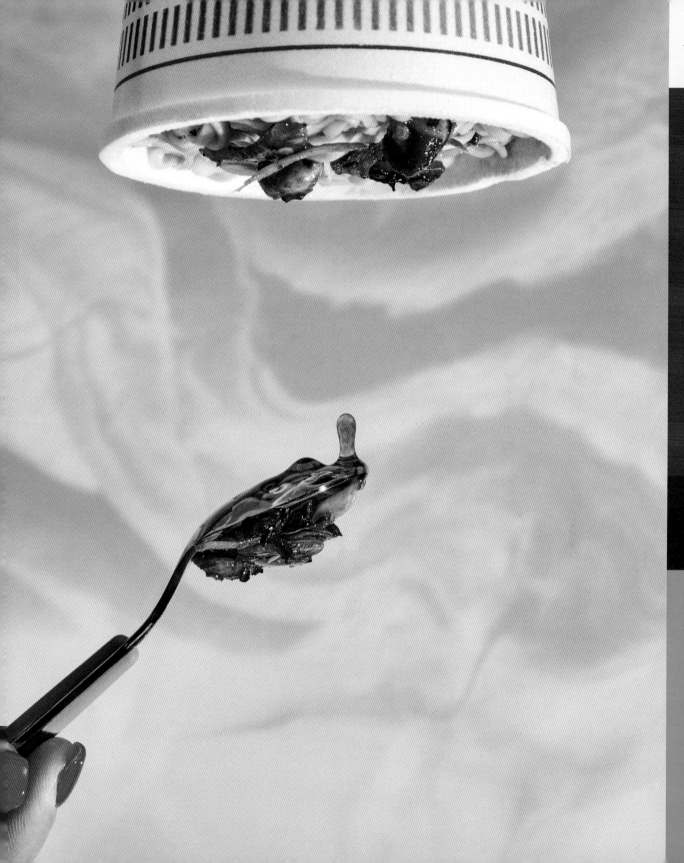

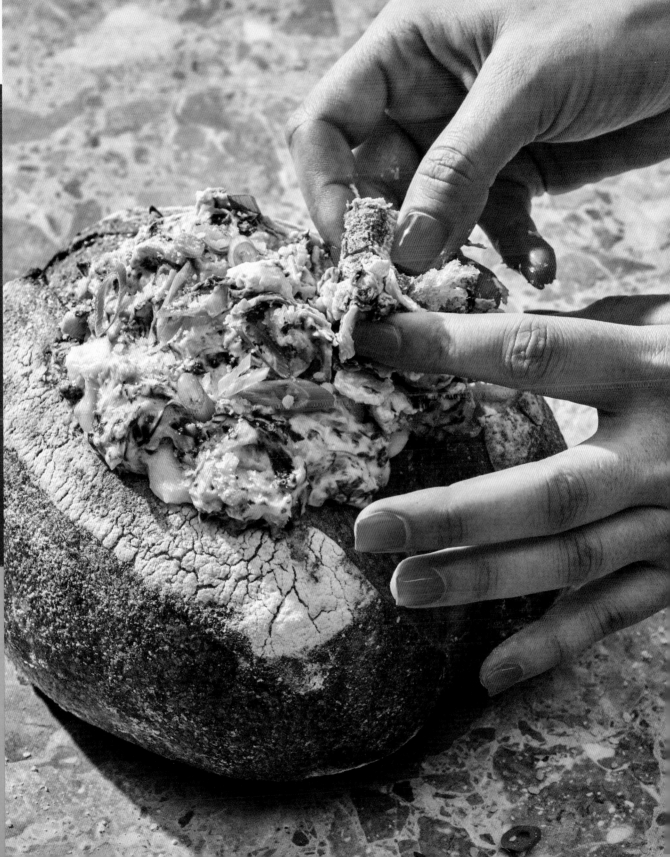

DOUBLE TRIP SPINACH DIP

SERVES 8

TIME: 30 minutes

DOSE: 6.25 mg THC
per ½ cup

Knorr spinach dip, served in a hollowed-out sourdough boule, starred at every family reunion, birthday, and holiday table. It was one of the first recipes my mom trusted me with, which isn't saying much, given how hard it is to mess up: Defrost the spinach, chop up the water chestnuts, combine the ingredients, and sprinkle with flavorful seasoning.

Nevertheless, I tinkered with the recipe by mixing the mayo and sour cream with the seasoning first, so the flavors evenly homogenize, and using the torn interior of the boule as a utensil to shovel the maltodextrin-laden dip into my mouth. As an adult, I still riff on the classic, but now I skip the Knorr seasoning in favor of a different flavor of greenery.

1   /   Preheat the broiler with a rack in the center.

2   /   Use a sharp knife to cut out a large circle from the top of the boule, while leaving an edge. Remove the top and pull out the inside of the bread, tearing it and the circular top into large bite-sized chunks. Set the boule and the bread bites aside.

3   /   In a medium sauté pan over medium-low heat, warm the olive oil. Add the garlic, scallion whites, and chili flakes and cook, stirring, until fragrant and bubbling, about 30 seconds. Stir in the flower, then add the spinach, a handful at a time, to help it wilt down. Season with the salt and continue cooking until most of the moisture in the spinach evaporates, about 5 minutes. Add the artichokes and scallion greens, then cook, stirring, for another 2 minutes.

4   /   Add the cream cheese and mozzarella and stir until the cheeses fully melt, about 2 minutes. Remove from the heat and stir in the sour cream and Parmesan cheese.

5   /   Place the cored-out boule on a sheet pan and spoon in the dip. Broil on high for 5 to 6 minutes, until the top turns golden brown. Serve immediately, with the bread pieces for dipping.

1 sourdough boule

¼ cup extra-virgin olive oil

2 cloves minced garlic

2 scallions, divided (whites minced, greens sliced on a bias)

½ teaspoon red chili flakes

¼ gram ground decarboxylated flower

1 pound fresh spinach, roughly chopped

½ teaspoon kosher salt

1 (14-ounce) can quartered artichoke hearts, drained and roughly chopped

1 cup (8 ounces) cream cheese

1 cup (4 ounces) shredded low-moisture mozzarella cheese

½ cup sour cream

1 cup (2 ounces) finely grated Parmesan cheese

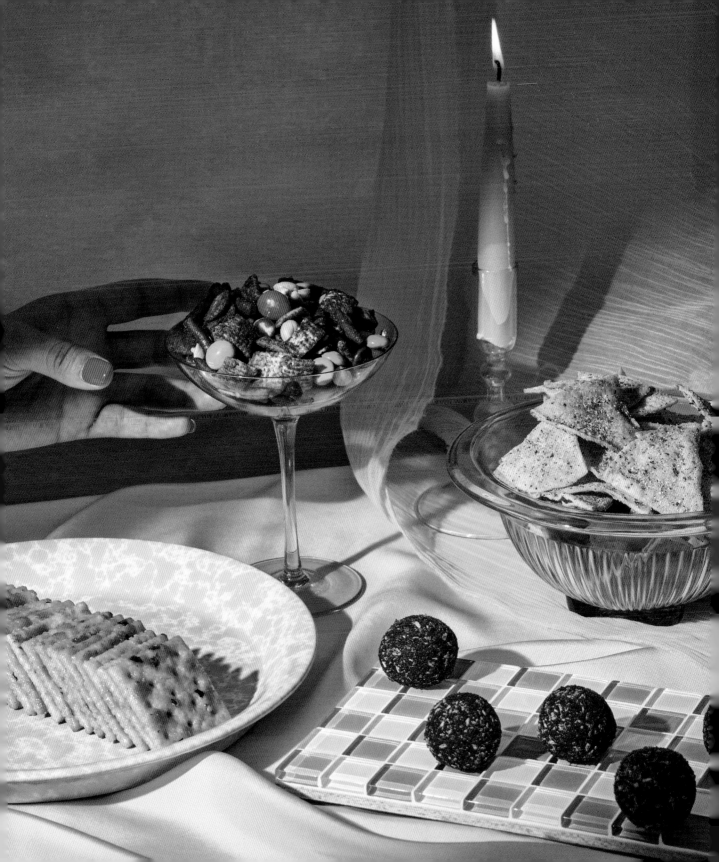

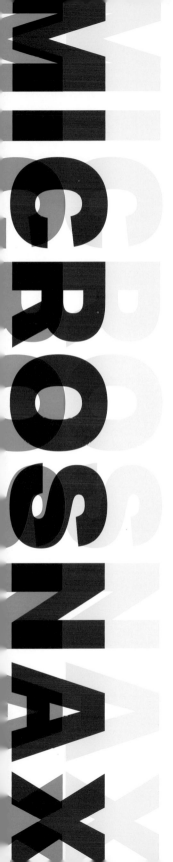

MICROSNAX

Buffer the day with a microdosed salty, crunchy, or chewy treat that satisfies a craving and takes the edge off. Whether you're on a leisurely stroll, stuck in boring meetings, or already melted into the couch, these gently dosed nibbles maintain the high.

CHILI RANCH TORTILLA CHIPS

SERVES 6 to 8

TIME: 50 minutes

DOSE: 2 mg THC
per chip

Inevitably, the spicy, cool seasoning on these chips sticks to your fingers, and I say, "Lick away." It's the best part! But the seasoning also carries the high, so be careful—and try to get an even sprinkle on each chip for a balanced dose.

1 / In a food processor, blend the ranch seasoning, Tajín, nutritional yeast, and flower until the weed mixes evenly throughout the flavor powder, about 30 seconds. Transfer to a small bowl and set aside.

2 / Cut each tortilla into 6 even triangles. Have a large bowl for tossing the chips ready. In a heavy-bottomed pot or Dutch oven over medium heat, bring the oil up to 350°F. Fry 4 to 6 tortilla triangles at a time, using a spider or slotted spoon to remove the tortillas when they turn a light brown, 3 to 5 minutes. Place in the large bowl and sprinkle 1 to 2 teaspoons of the seasoning mix over the handful of chips, tossing while they remain hot so the spices stick to the oil. Place the seasoned chips in a serving bowl and repeat with the remaining pieces of tortilla.

3 / Munch immediately.

1 (1-ounce) package ranch seasoning

1 tablespoon Tajín Clásico (chile-lime seasoning)

1 tablespoon nutritional yeast

½ gram ground decarboxylated flower

8 (6-inch) corn tortillas

3 cups neutral oil such as vegetable or canola for frying

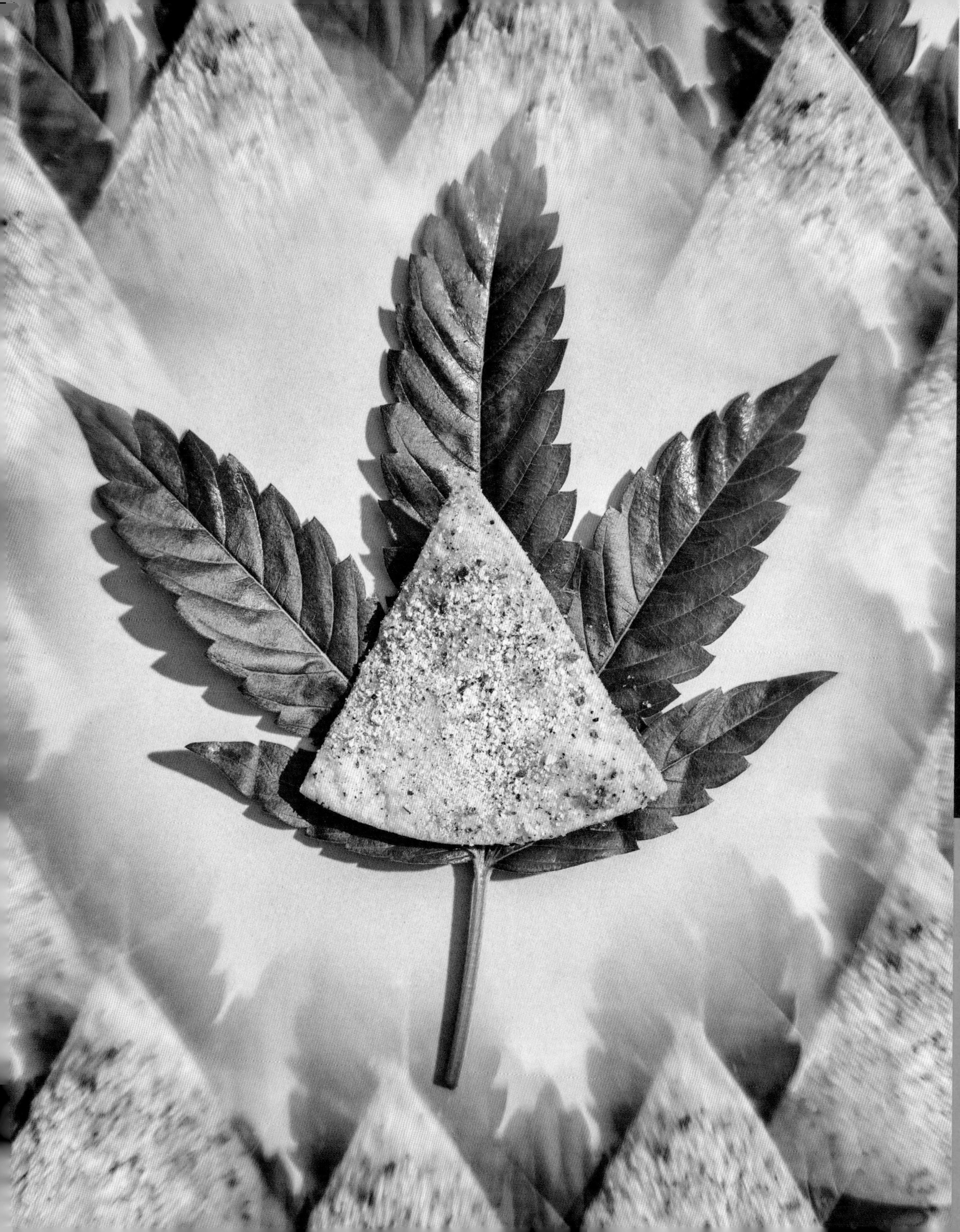

HEADS UP, POTHEAD!
Miso burns easily, so stay close to the
oven while baking.

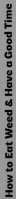

PARTY CRUNCH MIX

SERVES 24

TIME: 45 minutes

DOSE: 4 mg THC
per ½ cup

Some of the best stoner snacks come from religious zealots. Take graham crackers: The crunchy cookies started off as a healthy cracker developed by a reverend to help people abstain from earthly pleasures—long before anyone invented the s'more. Chex originates from a quirky New Age movement that preached temperance and a high-fiber diet. But my testament to the cult of snacks, a party mix that capitalizes on umami, worships only one thing: crunch.

1 / Preheat the oven to 325°F with a rack in the center.

2 / Line a sheet pan with parchment paper.

3 / In a 3-quart saucepan over low heat, melt both the butters, then add the maple syrup, miso, cinnamon, salt, and cayenne pepper and cook, stirring, for about 1 minute. Use a rubber spatula to stir everything together, then remove from the heat and set aside.

4 / In a large bowl, combine the cereal and both types of pretzels. Drizzle the miso-maple butter all over them and use a rubber spatula to toss it until the cereal is evenly coated. Spread the mix out on the sheet pan and bake, stirring every 10 minutes, for 30 to 35 minutes, until the miso-maple glaze takes on a caramel brown color and the cereal appears lightly toasted.

5 / Let the party mix cool completely, then transfer to a large bowl and add the nuts and both types of M&M's, tossing to mix.

6 / Enjoy immediately or store in a labeled airtight container for up to 2 weeks.

¼ cup (2 ounces) Cannabutter (page 61)

¼ cup (2 ounces) unsalted butter

½ cup maple syrup

⅓ cup white miso

1 tablespoon ground cinnamon

1 teaspoon kosher salt

¼ teaspoon ground cayenne pepper

6 cups (210 grams) Chex cereal

2 cups (120 grams) pretzel sticks, halved

2 cups (80 grams) mini pretzel twists

1 cup (165 grams) roasted salted mixed nuts

1 cup (235 grams) plain M&M's

1 cup (200 grams) peanut M&M's

TREEHUGGER GRANOLA

MAKES 9 cups

TIME: 1 hour

DOSE: 4 mg THC
per ½ cup

My senior year at Berkeley, I rocked a shaved head, smoked pinner joints walking across campus, and got really into edibles. I passed the activists camped out in the oak grove below the Greek theater as I walked to Telegraph Avenue to buy the dank snickerdoodles from the table covered with Bob Marley pins. I nibbled on the stale cookies while sitting through lectures on the differences between Monet and Manet, but they weren't exactly brain food. Having this edible ode to my time at Cal, packed with oats, nuts, and dried fruit, to snack on would have been far better. But que Seurat, Seurat.

1 / Preheat the oven to 325°F with a rack in the center. Line a sheet pan with parchment paper.

2 / In a large heat-safe bowl, combine the oats, coconut, and both nuts, then set aside.

3 / In a 3-quart saucepan over medium heat, combine the sugar, maple syrup, both butters, molasses, and salt. Use a rubber spatula to stir until the butters melt, 2 to 3 minutes. Stir the orange zest, cinnamon, and nutmeg into the butter mixture until the cinnamon is evenly distributed. Pour the mixture over the bowl of oats and nuts, using the spatula to scrape all the dosed syrup out of the saucepan. Stir and toss the granola to coat evenly, then pour onto the prepared sheet pan and spread out evenly.

4 / Bake for 15 minutes, then remove and stir, as the outside will cook faster than the inside. Bake for 25 to 30 more minutes, until the granola takes on a golden-brown color. Remove from the oven, stir in the dried cherries, and let cool, undisturbed—I like a few clusters, and this helps chunks stick together.

5 / Bag the granola for friends or store in a labeled airtight container in the pantry for 2 to 3 months.

3 cups (300 grams) old-fashioned rolled oats

1 cup (120 grams) shredded unsweetened coconut

⅔ cup (100 grams) roughly chopped raw almonds

⅔ cup (100 grams) whole raw cashews

½ cup (100 grams) granulated sugar

½ cup maple syrup

3 tablespoons (1½ ounces) Cannabutter (page 61)

5 tablespoons (2½ ounces) unsalted butter

2 teaspoons blackstrap molasses

1 teaspoon kosher salt

2 teaspoons grated orange zest (about 1 large orange)

1 teaspoon ground cinnamon

½ teaspoon ground nutmeg

⅔ cup (100 grams) dried cherries

CRACKED-UP CRACKERS

MAKES 150 crackers

TIME: 1 hour 40 minutes

DOSE: 1 mg THC per 3 crackers

You can have too much of a good thing, especially edibles. Stoner lore has long held that chewing black pepper changes the trajectory of a bad trip. The theory is that when beta-caryophyllene—the main terpene and dietary cannabinoid found in black pepper—combines with THC, it chills you out.

These cacio e pepe–inspired crackers combine a fun way to calm the F down with America's favorite Roman pasta. Each cracker contains less than half a milligram of THC, so guests can eat them by the handful. Just make sure to use freshly ground black pepper.

1 / In a food processor, combine the pecorino, cream cheese, cheddar, cannabutter, pepper, and salt and blend to a paste, about 2 minutes. Add the flour and pulse until a dough forms, about 15 pulses. On a floured surface, roll the dough into a 4-inch-long log, wrap in plastic, and refrigerate for an hour.

2 / Preheat the oven to 350°F.

3 / Remove the dough from the fridge and let it sit at room temperature while the oven warms.

4 / Place the dough on a silicone baking mat (preferred) or large piece of parchment paper, then place another large piece of parchment paper on top of the dough. Using a rolling pin, roll the dough into a 10 x 15-inch rectangle that's about ⅛ inch thick. Chill in the fridge for 5 minutes, then remove the top sheet of parchment. Using a knife, score the dough into 150 squares by making 10 horizontal lines and 15 vertical lines. Dot the center of each square with a paring knife.

5 / Transfer the silicone baking sheet or parchment paper to a sheet pan and bake until golden brown, 20 to 22 minutes. Remove from the oven and let cool for 2 minutes before breaking into pieces. Let cool on a wire rack; they will get crunchier.

6 / Serve immediately or store in a labeled airtight container at room temperature for 1 week or freeze for up to a month.

½ cup (1½ ounces) finely grated pecorino cheese

¼ cup (2 ounces) cream cheese

¼ cup (1 ounce) grated sharp white cheddar

2 tablespoons (1 ounce) Cannabutter (page 61)

1 tablespoon freshly ground black pepper

½ teaspoon kosher salt

½ cup (60 grams) all-purpose flour, plus more for dusting

BLISS BALLS

MAKES 22 balls

TIME: 18 minutes

DOSE: 1 mg THC
per ball

The combination of high-protein nuts and sweet dates in these microdosed balls can fuel workouts and elevate endurance. Contrary to the "lazy stoner" trope, exercising on edibles—whether a vigorous vinyasa or rhythmic lap swim—helps athletes tune out the noise and tune in to their bodies. When we exercise, we produce more of the endocannabinoid anandamide, known as the bliss molecule, which creates the runner's high. That's probably why a study of older adults at the University of Colorado Boulder found that the stoners of the bunch exercised more than those who pass on grass.

1 / In a food processor, pulverize the raspberries into a powder, about 1 minute. Scoop into a medium bowl, add the shredded coconut, and stir to combine. Tip the bowl out onto a sheet pan and set aside.

2 / In the now-empty food processor, combine the dates, walnuts, almonds, rolled oats, honey, cocoa powder, and salt and blend until the dates and nuts clump into a single mass, about 3 minutes. Use a rubber spatula to transfer the mixture into a medium bowl and stir to make sure the nuts are evenly mixed with the dates.

3 / Use a tablespoon measure to scoop a chunk of date mixture into your hands and roll it into a relatively smooth ball. Place the ball on the raspberry-and-coconut-covered sheet pan. Repeat with the remaining mixture until you have formed 22 balls. Roll the balls around on the sheet pan until they are evenly covered in pink coconut flakes.

4 / Bliss out immediately or store the balls in a labeled airtight container in the fridge for up to 2 weeks.

¼ cup freeze-dried raspberries

½ cup shredded unsweetened coconut

1½ cups Medjool dates (about 12)

¾ cup raw walnut halves

⅔ cup raw unsalted almonds

3 tablespoons rolled oats

¼ cup Whipped Weed Honey (page 78)

1 tablespoon Dutch-process cocoa powder

½ teaspoon kosher salt

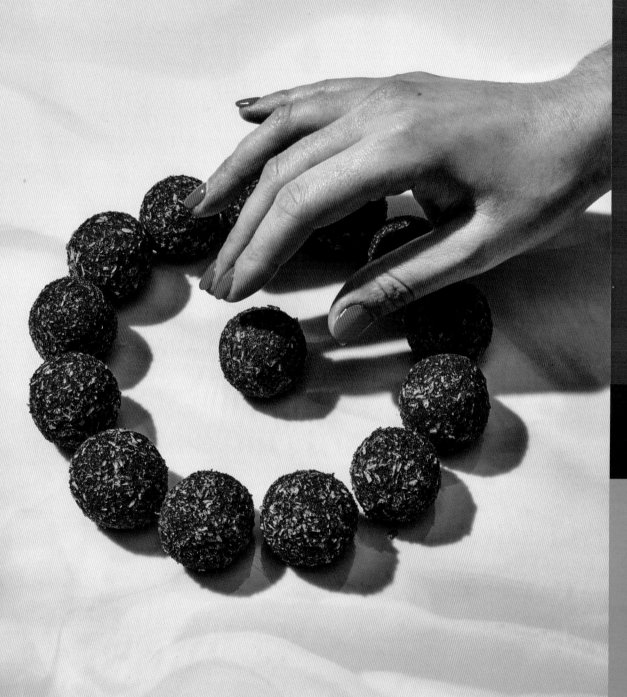

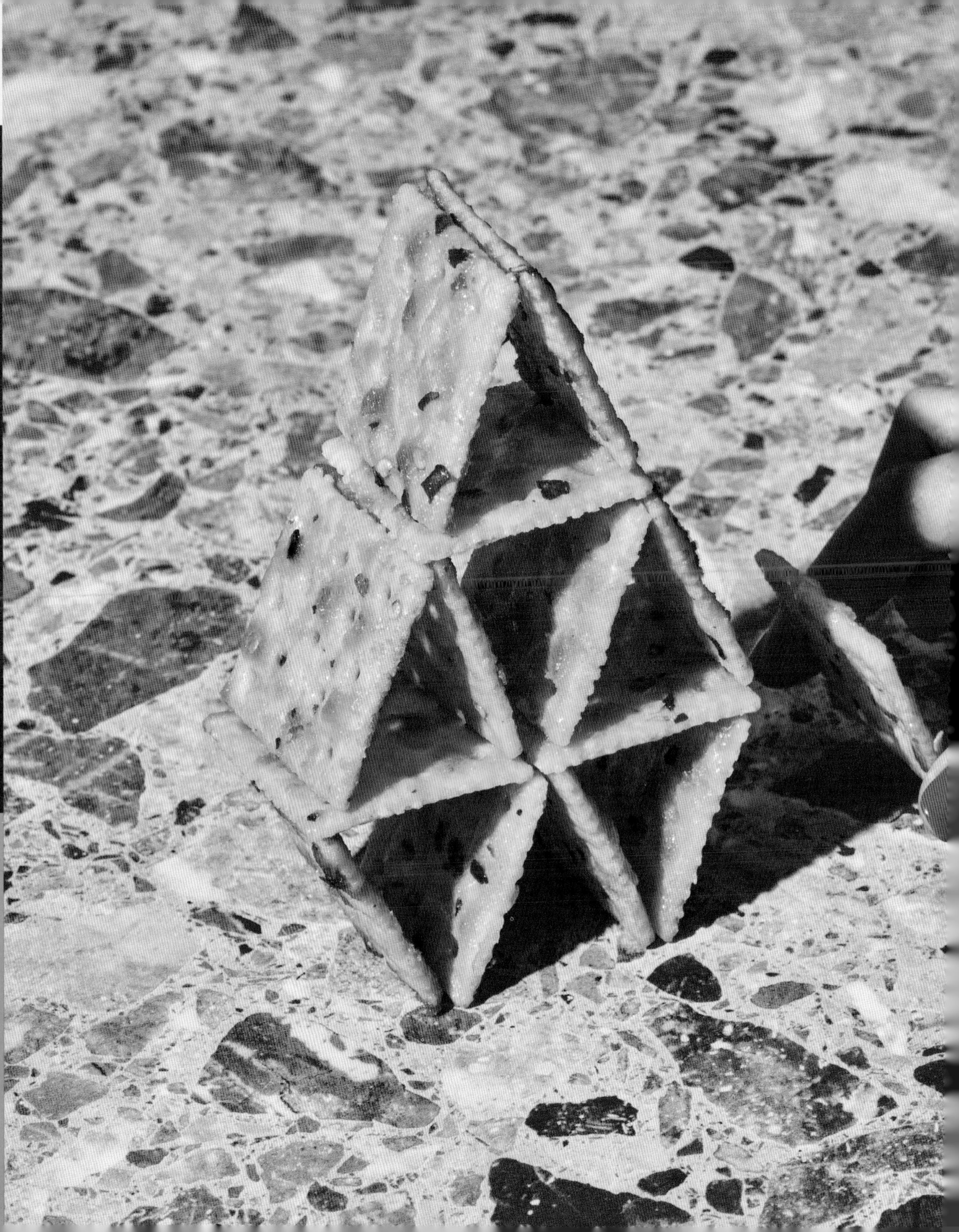

HOT HONEY FIRECRACKERS

MAKES 160
crackers

TIME: 20 minutes

DOSE: 1 mg THC
per 3 crackers

A top-tier snack needs sweetness, saltiness, a kick of heat, and lots of crunch. These put a twist on a Southern classic by swapping out ranch dressing for nutritional yeast and adding honey to balance the chili flakes. Traditional firecrackers soak the saltines in seasoned oil overnight, but this version switches the oil to melted butter, which contains water, so baking crisps up the crackers and shellacks the honey to their ridges.

1   /   Preheat the oven to 325°F and line two sheet pans with parchment paper.

2   /   In a medium saucepan over medium-low heat, melt both the butters. Remove from the heat and vigorously whisk in the honey, nutritional yeast, red chili flakes, and salt.

3   /   Place the saltines in a large resealable bag or big bowl and pour the infused honey butter over the crackers. Gently shake the bag or use a rubber spatula to toss them in the bowl to evenly coat the crackers.

4   /   Place half the batch of crackers in a single layer on the prepared sheet pans. Bake the crackers, flipping after 4 minutes, until the honey starts to caramelize and the crackers turn golden brown on each side, a total of 8 to 10 minutes. Transfer to a wire rack to cool. Repeat with the remaining crackers and let cool completely before munching.

5   /   Snack immediately or store in a labeled lidded container for up to a week.

¾ cup plus 2 tablespoons (7 ounces) unsalted butter

2 tablespoons (1 ounce) Cannabutter (page 61)

¼ cup honey

¼ cup nutritional yeast

1 tablespoon red chili flakes (adjust depending on heat preference)

½ teaspoon kosher salt

1 (16-ounce) package saltine crackers

WONDER-FULL PEANUT BUTTER PRETZELS

MAKES 24 pretzels

TIME: 2 hours 45 minutes

DOSE: 4 mg THC per pretzel

The secret to homemade pretzels is baked baking soda. Baked as in baked in the oven, not baked like me after I eat a quarter-batch of these crispy-chewy peanut-butter-and-white-chocolate-filled treats. Baking soda is made of sodium bicarbonate, and heating it turns it into sodium carbonate, a more alkalized salt that alters the pH balance and salinity of the water. Sodium carbonate gives these pretzels their chewy, salty exterior. Then, the super salty water tightens the gluten structure around the outside, leaving the inside soft, with a surprise in the center.

1 / Preheat the oven to 300°F.

2 / In the bowl of a stand mixer with the whisk attachment, combine the lukewarm water and 1 tablespoon of the molasses on low speed until the molasses dissolves in the water, about 1 minute. Sprinkle the yeast over the molasses water and whisk together for a few seconds. Sift both flours into the bowl, then add the cannabutter and kosher salt. Switch to the dough hook and mix on low speed for 2 minutes, then turn the speed up to medium-high until the dough is smooth and elastic, about 8 minutes. Scrape the sides with a rubber spatula, if needed, to make sure all the ingredients are incorporated. Grease a large bowl with the neutral oil, add the dough, cover with plastic wrap, and leave in a warm place to rise until at least double in size, about an hour.

3 / While the dough rises, prepare the filling: In a microwave-safe bowl, heat the white chocolate in the microwave in 15-second intervals, stirring in between, until completely melted, about 2 minutes total. Using a rubber spatula, stir the peanut butter into the chocolate until fully combined, then put the mixture in the freezer for 5 to 6 minutes to stiffen up. Line a sheet pan with parchment paper and use a teaspoon

⅔ cup lukewarm water

1 tablespoon plus 1 teaspoon blackstrap molasses, divided

1 teaspoon active dry yeast

1¼ cups (150 grams) all-purpose flour, plus more for dusting

1¼ cups (150 grams) bread flour

¼ cup (2 ounces) Cannabutter (page 61), room temperature

1 teaspoon kosher salt

1 teaspoon neutral oil such as vegetable or canola to grease the bowl

¼ cup (50 grams) white chocolate

½ cup creamy peanut butter

⅓ cup baking soda

1 large egg

1 tablespoon whole milk

¼ cup coarse sea salt

HEADS UP, POTHEAD!
This recipe gets a little complicated, so have (or be) a sober supervisor on hand.

measure to scoop 24 balls of the peanut butter mixture onto the sheet pan. Place the balls back in the freezer until the dough is ready.

4 / Spread the baking soda onto a sheet pan and bake for 30 minutes, stirring halfway through. Remove from the oven and set aside. The baking soda is highly alkaline, so avoid getting it on your skin.

5 / Turn the oven up to 350°F.

6 / When the dough doubles in size, punch it down and cover again with a damp kitchen towel or plastic wrap.

7 / In a medium pot over medium-high heat, add 6 cups of water, the baked baking soda, and remaining 1 teaspoon of molasses and bring to a boil.

8 / Sprinkle flour on the counter and tip the dough out, then pat the dough into a rectangle. Cut the dough into 4 rows by 6 rows to make 24 pieces. Remove the tray of peanut butter balls from the freezer. Use your hands to roll a piece of dough into a ball, then flatten into a disk. Place a frozen peanut butter ball in the center of the disk and quickly wrap the dough around the ball, pinching the seams. Place the finished pretzel ball on a sheet pan and repeat with remaining balls.

9 / Use a slotted spoon to add 6 pretzel balls at a time to the medium pot and boil for 3 minutes, then scoop out and place on a cooling rack. Repeat with the rest of the pretzel balls.

10 / In a small bowl, whisk together the egg and milk. Line two sheet pans with parchment paper. Place the boiled pretzels 3 by 4 on each pan. Brush with the egg wash and sprinkle with coarse sea salt. Bake for 15 to 16 minutes, until the outside turns shiny and a rich brown. Let cool on the pan for 5 to 6 minutes.

11 / Enjoy while still a little warm. Store in a labeled airtight container for 1 to 2 days.

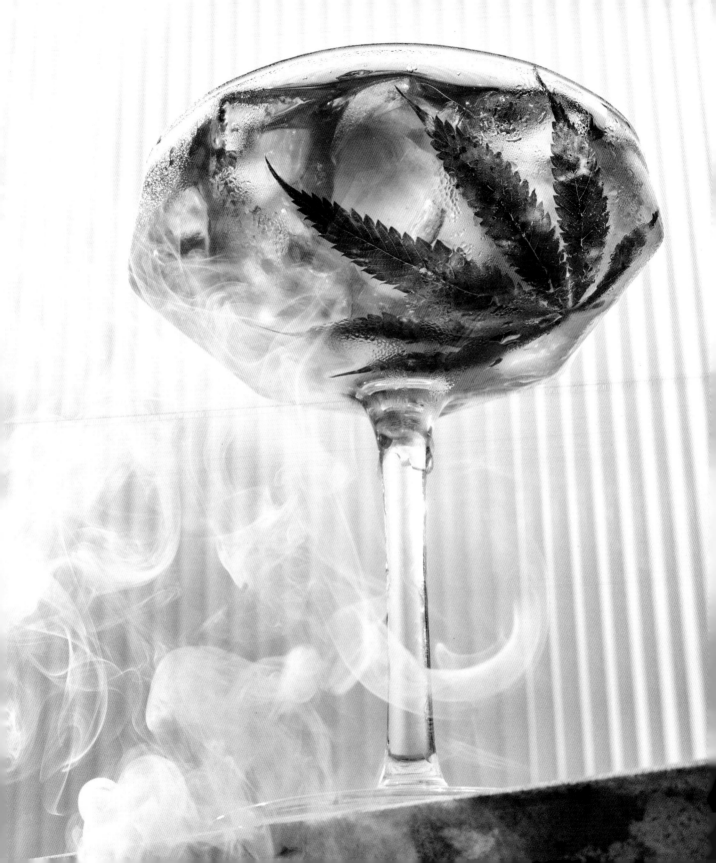

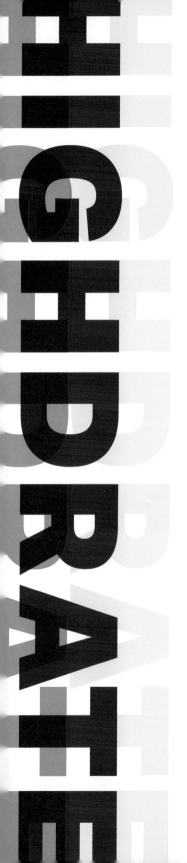

HIGHBRATE

Skip the alcohol—and the hangover—by spiking the party's punch with grass. Hot or cold, shaken or stirred, these lifted libations blend cannabis into delightfully potent potables. And, since our bodies digest liquids more easily than solids, their highs hit faster.

How Not to Crossfade

Being friends with a celebrity stylist means any bad moment becomes that much more mortifying—because you didn't just puke, you puked in the manicured rosemary bushes of a forever-young model-actress.

I met my stoner stylist friend on the set of *Paper* magazine's first food issue. I guest edited and he styled the chefs, butchers, and bakers. I picked him up from LAX with a rolled joint, ready to blaze before dinner at the Diesel store on Melrose. At dinner I ate a plate of lemon-dressed salmon, drank a few glasses of white wine and, perhaps, a Champagne or two; who can remember?

After dinner, we headed to a dimly lit, mahogany-wrapped bar, where I ordered a bourbon to drown my nerves before meeting his movie-star friend. I took a gulp, stepped onto the patio, and offered the starlet a spliff. I found myself clearing rips from a two-foot bong in her Los Feliz mansion not long after.

I started coughing from a hot rip and then felt the salmon jiggle in my stomach, so I walked outside to get some air. A few moments later, my friend held my hair back as I uncontrollably yakked in the English-style garden.

Depending on tolerance levels, individual biology, and countless other variables, everyone responds differently to both smoking and drinking. But research proves that I'm not the only one who has tossed their cookies after shots and pot: Mixing alcohol and weed makes almost everyone nauseated. Studies show that drinking alcohol before smoking weed increases the absorption of THC. For a seasoned stoner and drinker, this heightened effect might sound fun, but for most people, the mix isn't worth the risk.

Now I choose: either alcohol or weed (usually weed). Some of the drinks in this book contain a little bit of alcohol as a tincture or flavor component, but never enough to give a buzz. If crossfading still somehow sounds fun to you, try to smoke before drinking, as one study found that weed actually delays the intoxicating effects of alcohol. If only I knew that before I met my celebrity crush, I might have slipped her my number instead of slipping out without saying goodbye.

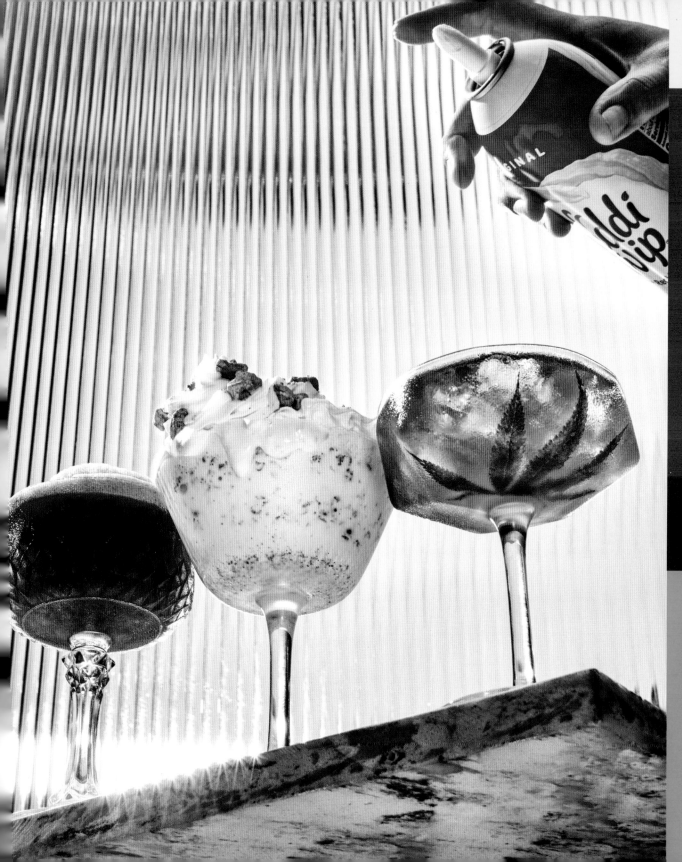

UNCLE NED'S WAKE AND SHAKE

SERVES 4

TIME: 5 minutes

DOSE: 3 mg THC
per smoothie

In the late 1960s, my uncle Ned opened Modo Natural Foods on Kauai, naming it after a word he found in *Autobiography of a Yogi*. The juice and smoothie store operated on what he called "a real hippy scale, back in the Summer of Love." He blended together produce from his macadamia farm in Lawai to make this smoothie—and he still does to this day.

His colony of bees feed on the seasonal floral blooms of the island, and he processes their honey in a small shack built out of an old guava tree, pouring it into mason jars to hand out to friends and family. But the real magic of Uncle Ned's smoothies comes from the creaminess of the macadamia nuts, the freshly squeezed citrus, and the total eschewing of fancy add-ins. He prefers tangy tangelo juice mixed with caramel-sweet Valencia oranges and a little bit of lime for tartness, but feel free to experiment with any variety of citrus—as long as it's freshly squeezed.

1 / In a blender, purée all of the ingredients together on high until smooth, about 2 minutes.

2 / Pour into tall glasses and enjoy immediately or refrigerate in a lidded container for up to 2 days.

2 cups freshly squeezed orange juice, about 8 oranges

1 large banana, frozen

2 cups crushed ice

½ cup macadamia nuts

2 tablespoons Whipped Weed Honey (page 78)

2 tablespoons freshly squeezed lime juice (about 1 lime)

HONEYDEW YOU SLUSHY

SERVES 6

TIME: 10 minutes

DOSE: 5 mg THC
per slushy

This drink leans heavily on the honeydew, so take the time to pick the right one. Picking a honeydew takes a level of intimacy with the melon: Look for a round, evenly colored fruit, then press lightly on the circle at the blossom end, opposite the stem, to gauge the ripeness of the inner flesh. Overripe honeydew pushes in like a deflated tennis ball; underripe stays firm. Look for tautness, but with slight give. Take a big whiff of both the blossom and stem end to check for a subtly floral honey aroma. Then use the melon to blitz up this slushy on a hot day and honeydew nothin'.

1 / In a blender, add the honeydew, lime juice, lime sherbet, mint, Turnt Tincture, and salt. Blend on low speed until the honeydew is fully blended and the mint turns to small specks, about 1 minute. Add the ice and blend on medium speed (or high speed, if needed) until the ice looks slushy, another 1 to 2 minutes.

2 / Pour into 6 tall glasses and garnish each with a sprig of mint. Serve with straws and slurp up immediately.

5 cups cubed honeydew melon
(about ½ a 5-pound melon)

½ cup freshly squeezed lime juice
(about 4 limes)

1 cup lime sherbet

⅓ cup fresh mint leaves, plus more
for garnish

½ tablespoon Turnt Tincture (page 70)

Pinch of fine sea salt

2 cups crushed ice

THE GRAPE BEYOND FIZZ

SERVES 4

TIME: 5 minutes

DOSE: 2.5 mg THC
per fizz

Just before I started selling hash caramels, a mixologist with a waxed mustache whipped up my first foamy egg white–crested cocktail at a bar called The Alembic in San Francisco. I sampled my syrupy drink from its dainty glass and planned my edibles enterprise. The crown of frothy, sugary egg whites intrigued me, demonstrating the intersection of confection and cocktail. The nostalgic Grape Beyond Fizz takes me back to sipping fancy drinks and dreaming up a world of cannabis cuisine. But instead of waking up hungover, I just close my eyes and drift into sweet dreams.

1 / In a cocktail shaker, add the grape juice, lemon juice, sugar, egg white, and ice, then shake vigorously to create a foam, about 30 seconds. Strain and pour the infused grape liquid evenly among 4 cocktail glasses, then finish with a splash of soda water. If any froth remains in the shaker, top off the glasses.

2 / Clink glasses and drink up.

¾ cup Concord grape juice

¼ cup freshly squeezed lemon juice (about 2 lemons)

1 tablespoon Stoned Sugar (page 77)

1 large egg white

¼ cup crushed ice

Splash of soda water, for finishing

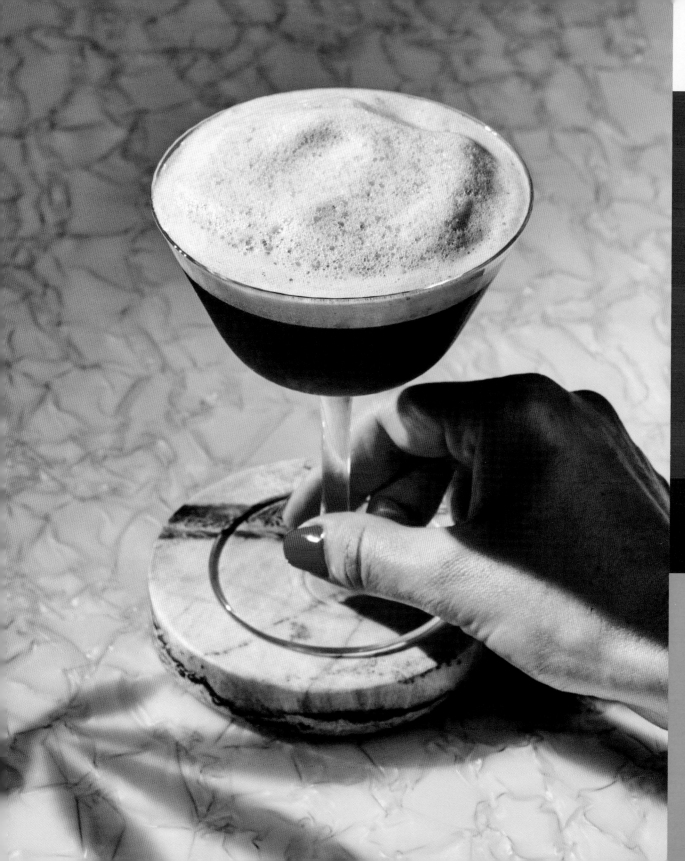

CHILLED-OUT ALMOND MOCHA

SERVES 4

TIME: 5 minutes

DOSE: 6.25 mg THC
per drink

Caffeine and weed have gone together since Amsterdam's cafes started offering lattes with a slice of space cake. Blend one of these caffeinated refreshers up on a midsummer afternoon and embrace the chill motivation throughout the rest of the day.

1 / If you made the fudge sauce ahead of time or refrigerated it, warm it up by microwaving it in 30-second intervals, stirring between each, until smooth and melted again, 2 to 3 minutes total.

2 / In a blender, pulse the milk, 5 tablespoons of the fudge sauce, the orgeat syrup, instant espresso powder, and almond extract until it looks like chocolate milk, about a minute. Add the ice and purée on low speed until all the ice in the frappé looks blended, 2 to 3 minutes (too high a speed will cause the ice to seize). Drizzle more fudge sauce along the interior sides of 4 clear glasses. Pour a cup of coffee slushy into each glass, top with whipped cream, drizzle with any remaining fudge, and sprinkle with almonds.

3 / Serve with straws and enjoy immediately.

½ cup Faded Sundae Fudge Sauce (page 234), divided

1½ cups almond milk

¼ cup orgeat syrup

1 tablespoon instant espresso powder

1 teaspoon almond extract

4 cups crushed ice

Canned whipped cream, for garnish

Toasted sliced almonds, for garnish

HEADS UP, POTHEAD!
A healthy dose of Faded Sundae Fudge Sauce (page 234) brings the high, so you will want to have that warmed up and ready before you get started.

SERVING SUGGESTION:
Double the dose by replacing the almond flavor of the orgeat syrup with the Whipped Weed Honey (page 78) and an additional half-teaspoon of almond extract.

CANNABIS CHAI

SERVES 6

TIME: 20 minutes

DOSE: 4 mg THC
per ½ cup

When I lived in Berkeley, I celebrated any small accomplishment with a walk to Vik's Chaat for their humongous dosa, tamarind-doused pani puri, and a hot cup of chai, served in a small metal cup. Inspired by that piping hot chai, this tea uses ingredients that balance the flavor and high of cannabis, specifically the beta-caryophyllene in the black pepper. It feels fitting: Indian food has a long history with cannabis. Bhang, a paste made from cannabis leaves and flowers, mixes effortlessly into saffron-spiced sweets and nutty drinks like thandai to commemorate the festival of colors, Holi.

1 / Using a mortar and pestle, crush the cardamom and fennel seeds into pieces. Add the cloves and peppercorns and use the pestle to smash a few times, crushing, but not grinding, to a powder. Repeat with the cinnamon sticks, anise, and ginger. Scoop everything into a small bowl and add the nutmeg.

2 / In a 3-quart saucepan over medium heat, bring the water to a boil. Add the tea bags and lower the heat to medium-low to steep the tea for 2 minutes, stirring occasionally. Pour in both milks and add the bowl of spice mixture. Stir constantly until a light, white foam forms on the top, 10 minutes. Add the sugar and stir to combine.

3 / Strain the chai through a fine-mesh sieve and sip while hot.

1 teaspoon green cardamom seeds

½ teaspoon fennel seeds

½ teaspoon whole cloves

½ teaspoon whole black peppercorns

2 small cinnamon sticks

3 star anise petals

1 teaspoon peeled and grated fresh ginger

½ teaspoon ground nutmeg

2 cups water

4 black tea bags

1¼ cups whole milk

¼ cup Mota Milk (page 66)

2 tablespoons granulated sugar

SERVING SUGGESTION:
Make this recipe with whole milk to help a friend-in-need who ate too much weed—the beta-caryophyllene neutralizes the high (see page 46). Or serve it with Stoned Sugar (page 77) to bump up the effects.

CEREAL CHILLER MILKSHAKE

SERVES 4

TIME: 5 minutes

DOSE: 6.25 mg THC
per shake

As adults, we have the power to replace the milk in a bowl of cereal with a milkshake. Swirling crushed Fruity Pebbles in a vanilla shake adds a tropical medley of nostalgic flavors that masks the dank flavor of Mota Milk. The sprinkle of smashed Lucky Charms gets a little bit chewy on top, becoming a magical stoner treat, and, thankfully, they sell the marshmallows separately now, so that pesky cereal doesn't get in the way of the fun parts.

1   /   In a blender, combine the ice cream and both milks, starting at low speed, then on high, until the milkshake fully mixes, 1 to 2 minutes. Incorporate the crushed Fruity Pebbles by pulsing for 2 seconds, repeating if not well-dispersed. Pour into 4 tall glasses and top each with a shot of whipped cream and a sprinkle of smashed Lucky Charms marshmallows.

2   /   Serve with a wide straw and a spoon for the marshmallows.

6 cups (3 pints) vanilla ice cream

¼ cup Mota Milk (page 66), chilled

¾ cup whole milk

1⅓ cups crushed Fruity Pebbles

Canned whipped cream, for garnishing

½ cup Lucky Charms marshmallows, smashed

Highdrate

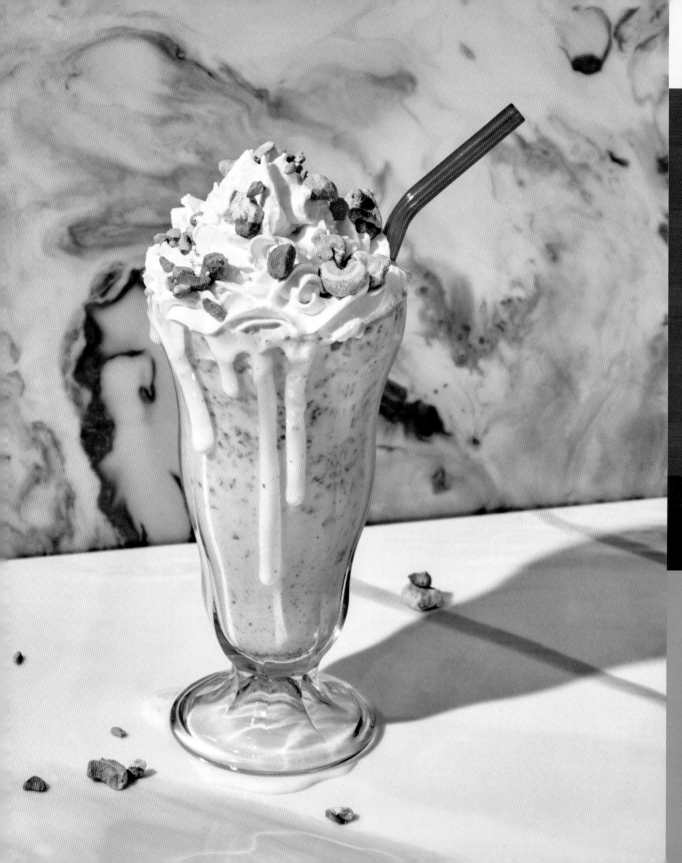

BONG ISLAND ICED TEA

SERVES 5

TIME: 20 minutes

DOSE: 6 mg THC
per cup

Long Island iced tea has five different types of booze, no tea, and an iconic reputation. People love the kitchen-sink drink because it gets them blitzed in a hurry, which makes it ripe for a stoner riff. This bubbly beverage contains actual tea, zero types of booze, and an upgrade to the original with a caffeine-and-cannabis combo. It tastes a lot like the cola gummies I bought at the concession stand as a kid: a little bit fizzy and slightly sweet, with a hint of tart.

1 / In a small saucepan or kettle, bring the water to a boil. Remove from the heat, add the tea bags, and steep in the hot water for 3 to 4 minutes. Discard the tea bags, pour the tea into a large jar or cup, and let the hot tea cool in the fridge before using, about 10 minutes.

2 / In a pitcher, stir together the cooled tea, Coca-Cola, ginger beer, lime juice, Turnt Tincture, and bitters until fully combined. Set out 5 glasses, fill with ice, and pour the tea mixture over it. Top each glass with a few sprigs of mint and a slice of lemon.

3 / Serve and enjoy.

2 cups water

2 black tea bags

2 cups Coca-Cola

½ cup ginger beer

½ cup freshly squeezed lime juice (about 4 limes)

½ tablespoon Turnt Tincture (page 70)

5 to 10 dashes of orange bitters

Fresh mint, for garnish

Sliced lemon, for garnish

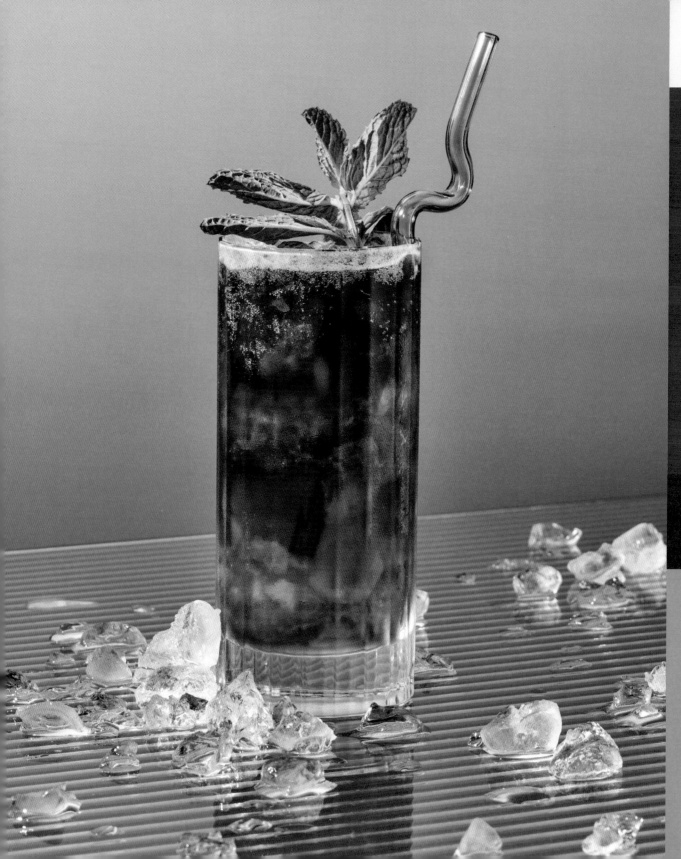

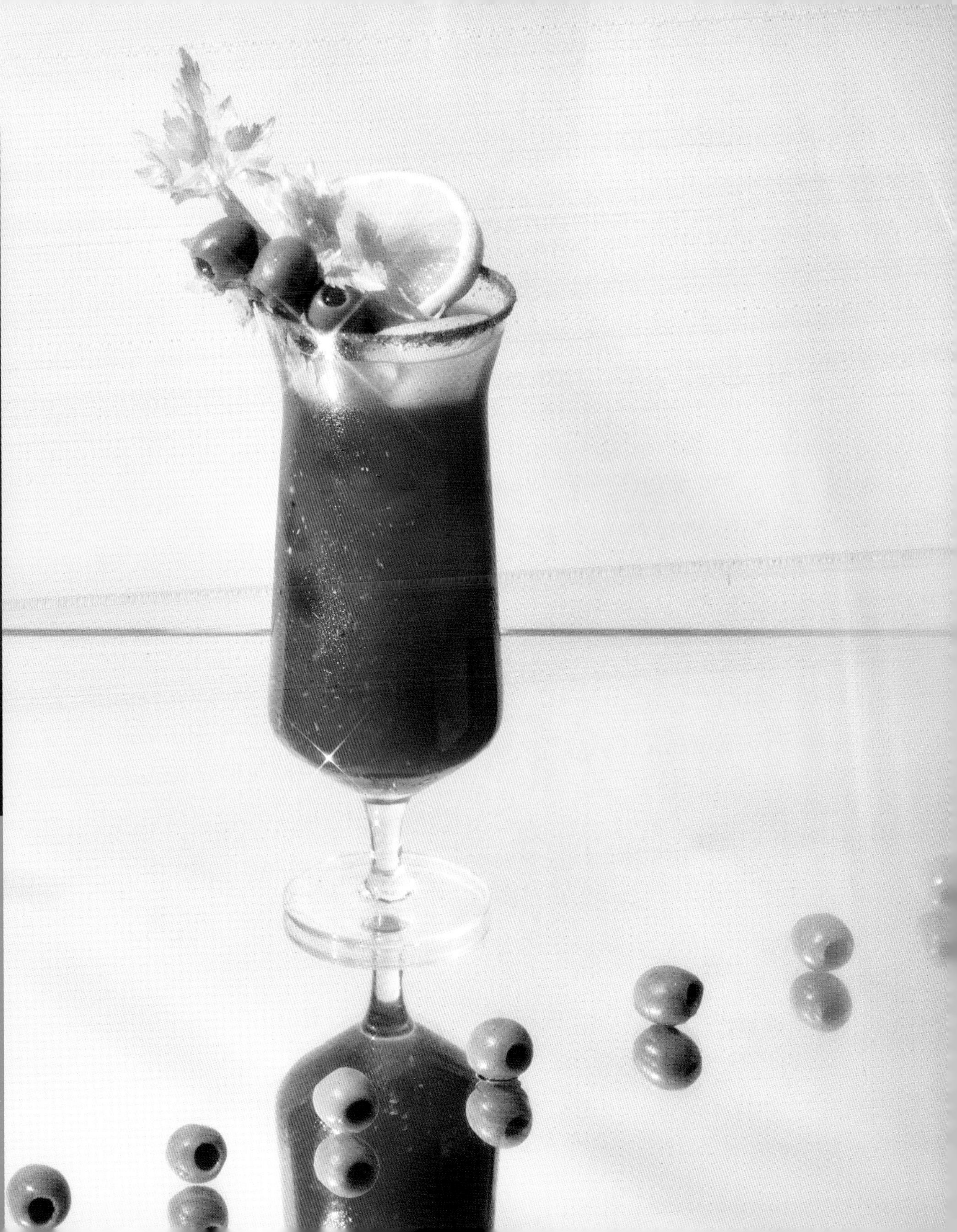

BLOODY MARY JANE

SERVES 6

TIME: 5 minutes

DOSE: 5 mg THC
per drink

I get a thrill out of drinks that come with snacks, and a classic Bloody Mary technically counts as a drinkable salad with a buzz at the end. This mix skips the booze in favor of a potent cannabis tincture, as I advise against crossfading (see page 144). But I do recommend extra olives, bacon, or blue cheese to intercept the munchies.

1 / In a large pitcher, combine the tomato juice, lemon juice, Worcestershire sauce, Turnt Tincture, prepared horseradish, pepper, hot sauce, and celery salt. Stir together until the horseradish fully blends into the mixture. Add a cup of ice, then stir again. Taste for spiciness and add more hot sauce, if desired. In each glass (I like to use mason jars), place ½ cup of ice, then pour the Bloody Mary Jane over the ice, splitting it evenly among the glasses. Poke 3 olives onto a toothpick and add to the glass along with a celery stick. Place a slice of lemon on the rim and a straw in the drink. Repeat with the remaining glasses.

2 / Drink right away, before the melting ice dilutes it.

6 cups tomato juice

⅓ cup freshly squeezed lemon juice (about 3 lemons)

¼ cup Worcestershire sauce

½ tablespoon Turnt Tincture (page 70)

¼ cup prepared horseradish

1 tablespoon freshly ground black pepper

1 tablespoon Louisiana-style hot sauce (such as Crystal or Tabasco), plus more to taste

1 teaspoon celery salt

4 cups cubed ice, divided

18 pimiento-stuffed olives

6 celery sticks

6 lemon slices

POT-A COLADA

SERVES 4

TIME: 5 minutes

DOSE: 6.25 mg THC
per colada

Literally "strained pineapple" in Spanish, the piña colada contains all the elements required for a tasty edible. First and foremost, fat, and lots of it, in the form of coconut milk. Then a bright flavor to dominate the palate: enter pineapple. Just make sure to use the sweetened cream of coconut, not unsweetened coconut cream, to bring it together into a refreshing cocktail that packs a potent dose.

1 / In a blender, combine the pineapple juice, pineapple chunks, cream of coconut, both coconut milks, lime juice, molasses, salt, and ice. Blend, starting on low speed for 1 minute, then increase to high and continue to blend until totally smooth, 2 to 3 minutes more. Stop and stir if the mixture gets stuck.

2 / Pour into 4 hurricane glasses, and place a pineapple wedge on each rim and a maraschino cherry on top. Serve with a straw and drink slowly to avoid brain freeze.

2½ cups pineapple juice

1 cup (140 grams) frozen pineapple chunks

½ cup cream of coconut

¼ cup coconut milk

¼ cup Mota Coconut Milk (page 66)

¼ cup freshly squeezed lime juice (about 2 limes)

1 teaspoon blackstrap molasses

Pinch of kosher salt

5 cups ice cubes

Fresh pineapple slices, for garnish

Maraschino cherries, for garnish

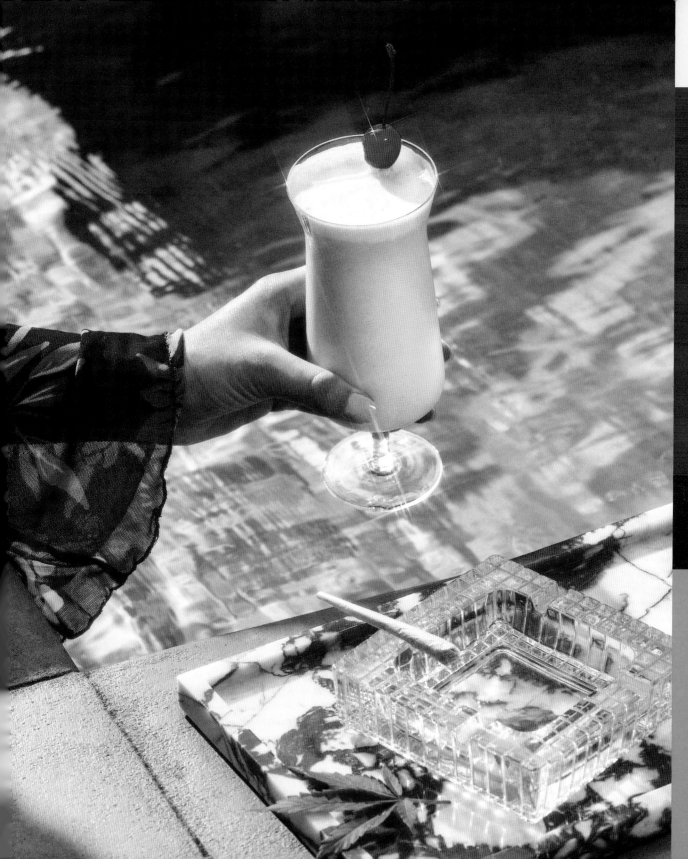

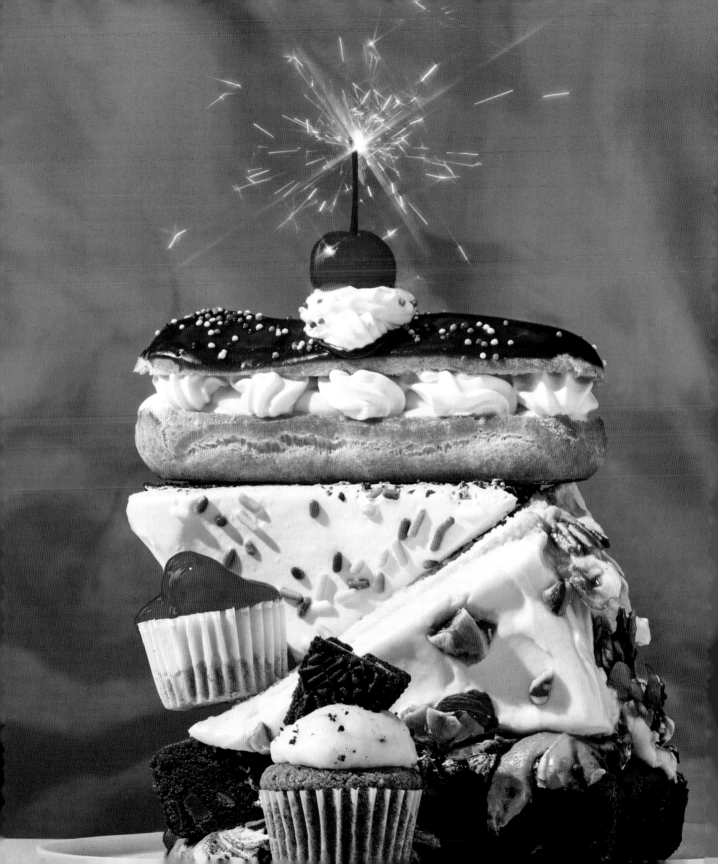

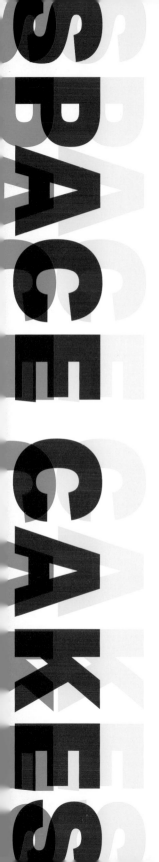

SPACE CAKES

Baking lifts spirits. Throw weed into the mix and get ready for takeoff. But skip the flight to Amsterdam and trip at home by creating your own celestial cake. Dosed desserts work well because sugar balances the bitterness of weed and most sweet treats call for a generous amount of fat, which makes infusion a snap.

BLUEST BLUEBERRY MUFFINS

MAKES 24 muffins

TIME: 50 minutes

DOSE: 4 mg THC
per muffin

After smoking a joint of Blueberry Kush and eating through a value pack of muffins from Costco, I had a stoner thought. Chocolate chip muffins become double-chocolate muffins with both a chocolate batter and chocolate chips, so why not apply the same logic to blueberry muffins? Having given it a try, I vote for more blueberries—in my weed and my muffins.

FOR THE CRUMBLE TOP

1 / In a small bowl, use a spoon to stir together the butter, both sugars, and salt. Add the flour and stir or use fingers to pinch the dough until it looks crumbly, with some bigger and smaller chunks of sugary butter. Set aside.

FOR THE MUFFINS

2 / Preheat the oven to 375°F with a rack in the center. Line a muffin tin (or two, adding up to 24 muffins total) with baking cups.

3 / In a large bowl, use a rubber spatula to combine the jam, milk, lemon zest, and vanilla extract. In a food processor, purée 1 cup of blueberries for just a few seconds, then stir into the jam-milk mixture.

4 / In a second large bowl, use a handheld mixer on medium speed to cream both butters with the sugar until light and fluffy, about 1 minute. Add the first egg, mix on high speed for several seconds, then add the second egg. Use a rubber spatula to scrape down the sides, then continue mixing until the batter turns light yellow, 30 seconds.

5 / In a medium bowl, whisk together 2½ cups flour, the baking powder, and the salt. Add about a third of the dry ingredients to the butter-egg bowl, using the spatula to stir in, but stop before they completely incorporate. Then add half of the blueberry-milk mixture, folding a few times. Repeat with another third of the dry ingredients and the rest of the blueberry-milk mixture, then the remaining dry ingredients. Stir until the batter looks cohesive and the flour disappears.

FOR THE CRUMBLE TOP

½ cup (4 ounces) unsalted butter, room temperature

⅓ cup (67 grams) granulated sugar

¼ cup (50 grams) dark brown sugar

Pinch of kosher salt

1¼ cups (180 grams) all-purpose flour

FOR THE MUFFINS

½ cup (150 grams) blueberry jam

¼ cup whole milk

1 teaspoon grated lemon zest
(½ large lemon)

1 teaspoon vanilla extract

3 cups (1 pound) blueberries, divided

¼ cup (2 ounces) Cannabutter (page 61), room temperature

¼ cup (2 ounces) unsalted butter, room temperature

1¼ cups (250 grams) granulated sugar

2 large eggs

2½ cups (300 grams) all-purpose flour, plus 1 tablespoon for coating blueberries

2 teaspoons baking powder

½ teaspoon kosher salt

6 / Add the remaining tablespoon of flour to the remaining 2 cups of blueberries, tossing to coat. Add the blueberries to the batter and fold one or two times to distribute. Spoon the batter into the prepared muffin tin, filling each cup two-thirds of the way up. Top each muffin with a heaping tablespoon of the crumble.

7 / Bake the muffins for 24 to 28 minutes, until the top turns a light golden brown and bounces back when lightly touched.

8 / Let cool on a wire rack for 15 minutes before eating. Store in a labeled lidded plastic container for 2 to 3 days.

CHOCOLATE CHIPS A'HIGH COOKIES

MAKES 36 cookies

TIME: 1 hour 30 minutes

DOSE: 5.5 mg THC per cookie

I make chocolate chip cookies more than any other recipe. It was the first cookie recipe I learned, and it gets better every time. The most important upgrade comes from eliminating brown sugar. As a kid, I hated the butt of dried-out bread my mom kept in the bag to keep the brown sugar moist. Now I use molasses instead of brown sugar in most of my baking, and it gives these classic chocolate chip cookies crispy edges and ooey-gooey insides.

Freezing the dough allows the butter to solidify, so the cookies spread less during baking and stay chewier. But it also ensures I have a freezer full of dough that I can bake into one or two cookies at a time.

1 / In a medium bowl, whisk together the flour, baking soda, and salt and set aside.

2 / Using a handheld mixer on medium speed, cream both butters with the sugar and molasses, scraping down the sides as needed, until the butter looks lighter in color and fluffy, 2 to 3 minutes. Turn the speed to low and add the first egg, beating until it is fully mixed in before adding the second. Stop as soon as the eggs disappear, about 1 minute. Add the vanilla and beat for another 30 seconds.

3 / Use a rubber spatula to fold in the dry ingredients, scraping the bottom, until just a few streaks of flour remain. Add the chocolate chips and give the batter several big stirs, so the chocolate chips are evenly distributed and the flour vanishes. Pop the dough in the fridge to stiffen up, about 30 minutes.

3 cups (360 grams) all-purpose flour

1 teaspoon baking soda

1 teaspoon kosher salt

½ cup (4 ounces) Cannabutter (page 61), room temperature

½ cup (4 ounces) unsalted butter, room temperature

2 cups (400 grams) granulated sugar

2 tablespoons blackstrap molasses

2 large eggs, room temperature

1 tablespoon vanilla extract

2 cups (12 ounces) bittersweet chocolate chips

4 / Use a tablespoon to scoop 36 heaping mounds of cookie dough onto a parchment-paper-lined sheet pan. Freeze the cookies on the pan for at least 30 minutes before baking. To store frozen, transfer to a labeled freezer bag and keep for up to 6 months.

5 / Center two racks in the oven and preheat the oven to 350°F.

6 / Line two sheet pans with parchment paper and place 18 dough lumps on each pan, spacing 1½ inches apart. Bake for 14 to 16 minutes, until the edges turn golden brown. Use a spatula to transfer to a wire rack and let cool for 1 or 2 minutes.

7 / Enjoy the cookies right away with a glass of cold milk or store in a labeled airtight container at room temperature for up to 3 days.

FUDGY FLUFFERNUTTY BROWNIES

MAKES 16 brownies

TIME: 1 hour 45 minutes

DOSE: 6.25 mg THC per brownie

Yes, I smoked a lot of pot before coming up with swirling peanut butter and Marshmallow Fluff on top of a bittersweet fudgy brownie. This mash-up bakes the classic pot brownie and kid-favorite fluffernutter sandwich together in a 9-inch baking pan. The ratio of sugar to flour in a brownie makes the difference between a cakey, dry square and an ooey-gooey morsel. The addition of molasses gives these brownies a moist, fudgy crumb, a heavy dose of sugar achieves the elusive chew, and the low-and-slow baking caramelizes the edges.

1 / Preheat the oven to 350°F with a rack in the center.

2 / Line a 9-inch square baking pan with parchment paper in both directions, leaving the edges hanging over the sides.

3 / In a large mixing bowl, pour the hot cannabutter over the chocolate and stir with a rubber spatula until the chocolate melts, 1 to 2 minutes. Add the molasses, salt, and vanilla extract, then mix thoroughly and set aside.

4 / In the bowl of a stand mixer fitted with the whisk attachment, beat the eggs on medium speed. Slowly add the sugar, whisking until the mixture quadruples in size, turns light yellow, and gets fluffy, 2 to 3 minutes.

5 / In a small bowl, whisk together the flour and cocoa powder.

6 / Use a rubber spatula to fold the chocolate-butter mixture into the eggs. When only a few streaks of egg remain, add the dry ingredients, folding until the flour just disappears. Pour into the lined pan, spreading evenly with the spatula.

7 / Lightly oil a small spoon and use it to drop Marshmallow Fluff on the top of the brownie batter in 4 rows of 4 dots each (each dot will

⅓ cup (2⅔ ounces) Brown Cannabutter (page 62), either still hot from preparation or reheated

¾ cup (4½ ounces) bittersweet chocolate chips

1 tablespoon blackstrap molasses

½ teaspoon kosher salt

1 tablespoon vanilla extract

3 large eggs

2 cups (400 grams) granulated sugar

¾ cup (90 grams) all-purpose flour

½ cup (45 grams) unsweetened Dutch-process cocoa powder

Neutral oil such as vegetable or canola, for greasing spoon

¼ cup Marshmallow Fluff

2 tablespoons creamy peanut butter

recipe continues

How to Eat Weed & Have a Good Time

be about ¾ teaspoon). Repeat with the peanut butter (each dot will be about ⅓ teaspoon) in between the rows of Fluff. Using a toothpick, swirl the Fluff and peanut butter in figure-eight motions throughout the batter to create an attractive Florentine pattern.

8 / Bake for 28 to 30 minutes, until the center registers 195°F on a thermometer or the top begins to crack and becomes shiny. Transfer the pan to a cooling rack and let the brownies cool in the pan for 15 minutes. Remove the brownies from the pan using the parchment paper overhang and let cool for 30 minutes on the rack. Cut the brownies into 16 even squares.

9 / Serve while still warm. Store in a labeled airtight container, with parchment paper separating any layers, for up to a week at room temperature, or wrap each brownie in plastic and then tinfoil, then label and freeze for up to 2 months.

ILLEGALLY BLONDIES

MAKES 16 blondies

TIME: 1 hour 10 minutes

DOSE: 6.25 mg THC per blondie

In high school, I worked at See's Candies. I wore a starched white button-up dress with a big black bow, gift wrapped boxes, and stuffed my face with chocolates. See's allowed their employees to eat as many chocolates as they wanted during their two fifteen-minute breaks. As a hormonal teenager, I took advantage of that perk daily. Eventually, I made myself sick enough that I cut down my sweet indulgence to only my favorite confections. To this day, the butterscotch square—basically brown sugar fudge coated in milk chocolate—ranks number one. These blondies, packed with blackstrap molasses and a hit of espresso, remind me of those squares, right down to the sugar high.

1   /   Preheat the oven to 350°F. Line a 9-inch square cake pan with parchment paper, leaving 2 inches of overhang in each direction.

2   /   In a large bowl, use a handheld mixer to blend together both butters, sugar, molasses, espresso powder, vanilla extract, and salt. Crack 1 egg into the bowl and mix until it all disappears into the batter, then add the second egg and continue beating for at least 30 seconds. Sift the flour and baking powder into the bowl and use a rubber spatula to gently fold the flour into the batter until no streaks remain. Take extra care to scrape the bottom; flour likes to hide below the batter.

3   /   Pour the batter into the prepared pan and spread evenly. Bake for 40 to 45 minutes, until the outside caramelizes and the top looks shiny, rather than wet.

4   /   Sprinkle the flaky sea salt on top and let cool in the pan on a wire rack for at least 15 minutes before cutting into 16 squares.

5   /   Enjoy right away or store in an airtight container for 2 to 3 days.

½ cup (4 ounces) unsalted butter, room temperature

⅓ cup (2⅔ ounces) Brown Cannabutter (page 62)

2 cups (400 grams) granulated sugar

¼ cup blackstrap molasses

2 tablespoons instant espresso powder

2 teaspoons vanilla extract

½ teaspoon kosher salt

2 large eggs

2 cups (240 grams) all-purpose flour

½ teaspoon baking powder

1 teaspoon flaky sea salt, such as Maldon

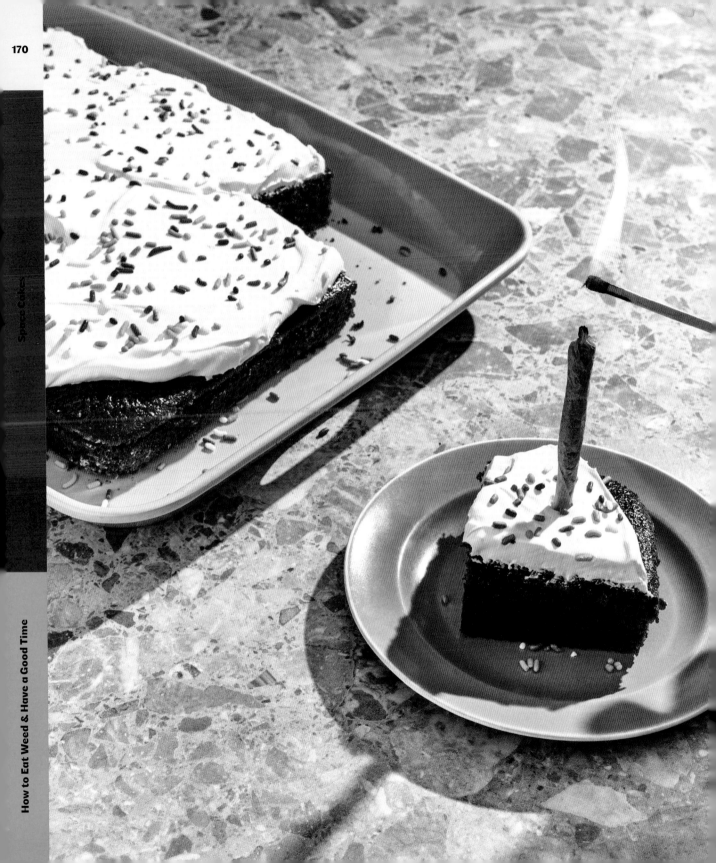

LIL' NESSA'S SNACK CAKE

MAKES 24 cakes

TIME: 2 hours

DOSE: 5 mg THC
per piece

In 1991 Little Debbie launched her cakes into outer space. Today, we can explore the galaxy from the comfort of the couch with a piece of this lifted chocolate cake, dolloped with Kewl Whip frosting, guaranteeing a blast whenever we want.

FOR THE CAKE

1 / Preheat the oven to 350°F with a rack in the center. Grease a 9 x 13-inch metal cake pan with butter and coat the pan with a tablespoon of cocoa powder.

2 / In a large bowl, sift together the remaining cocoa powder, cake flour, salt, baking soda, and baking powder. Whisk in the sugar.

3 / In a separate medium bowl, whisk together the milk, yogurt, eggs, and vanilla extract. Pour the wet ingredients into the dry, add both the oils and the hot water, then whisk everything together until the batter is completely smooth, about 1 minute.

4 / Pour the batter into the prepared pan and bake for 33 to 35 minutes, until a toothpick comes out clean or the top bounces back when pressed with a finger. Let cool completely in the pan on a wire rack for about an hour.

FOR THE FROSTING

5 / In a large bowl, whisk together the pudding mix and milk, then leave it to thicken for 5 minutes. Use a rubber spatula to fold in both the whips, then chill in the fridge for at least an hour. Dollop the frosting all over the cooled cake, using the back of a spoon to make dips and flips, then top with sprinkles. Slice in 4 rows by 6 columns to make 24 squares of snack cake.

6 / Enjoy the cake whenever. Store in a labeled lidded container in the fridge for up to 3 days.

FOR THE CAKE

Unsalted butter, for greasing

½ cup (45 grams) Dutch-process cocoa powder, plus 1 tablespoon for the pan

2 cups (240 grams) cake flour

1 teaspoon kosher salt

1 teaspoon baking soda

½ teaspoon baking powder

2 cups (400 grams) granulated sugar

½ cup whole milk

½ cup plain whole milk yogurt

2 large eggs

2 teaspoons vanilla extract

¼ cup neutral oil

¼ cup OOO Neutral Oil (page 64)

1 cup hot water

FOR THE FROSTING

1 (3.3-ounce) package vanilla pudding mix

¾ cup whole milk

1½ cups Cool Whip

1 cup Kewl Whip (page 198)

Rainbow sprinkles, for decoration

NOMNOM NANAIMO BARS

MAKES 16 bars

TIME: 2 hours

DOSE: 6.25 mg THC
per bar

Kids called me "Canada" when I went to high school in California, because I grew up in Alberta. But my upbringing means I am versed in the triple-layer, no-bake bars from the British Columbian city of Nanaimo. The key to the rich vanilla buttercream center comes from a quaint British product (and reminder of Canada's connection to the Commonwealth) called custard powder. The most common brand found in "the States" (as we say up north) is the delightfully old-school Bird's. But the secret to this version of a Nanaimo bar comes from the cannabutter woven through the fudgy coconut and almond crunch at the bottom.

1 / Line an 8-inch square cake pan with two pieces of parchment paper, one going in each direction, with some overhang on the sides for easy removal.

2 / Make a double boiler by filling a 3-quart saucepan with 2 cups of water and placing a medium metal bowl on top. Set the double boiler over medium-low heat. In the bowl, whisk together the cannabutter, ¼ cup of the unsalted butter, the granulated sugar, cocoa powder, egg, vanilla extract, and ¼ teaspoon of the salt. Cook, stirring, until the mixture thickens and turns shiny, 1 to 2 minutes. Remove from the heat and use a rubber spatula to stir in the graham cracker crumbs, coconut, walnuts, and almonds until well combined, then tip the mixture into the prepared baking pan. Press the mixture into the pan and use the flat bottom of a cup to press down and level the top. The goal is flat and even layers, to make sharp lines that highlight a drastic contrast between each section. Put the pan in the fridge to cool for at least 10 minutes while you prepare the next layer.

3 / In a medium bowl, use a handheld mixer on medium speed to cream together ¼ cup of the unsalted butter, the whipping cream, custard powder, powdered sugar, and the remaining ¼ teaspoon of salt. Beat until smooth and slightly fluffy, 1 to 2 minutes.

¼ cup (2 ounces) Cannabutter (page 61)

¾ cup (6 ounces) unsalted butter, room temperature, divided

⅓ cup (68 grams) granulated sugar

¼ cup (23 grams) Dutch-process cocoa powder

1 large egg

1 teaspoon vanilla extract

½ teaspoon kosher salt, divided

1 cup (142 grams) graham cracker crumbs (about 9 crackers)

1 cup (100 grams) unsweetened shredded coconut

¼ cup (30 grams) roughly chopped walnuts

¼ cup (35 grams) roughly chopped almonds

¼ cup heavy whipping cream

¼ cup (40 grams) custard powder

2 cups (240 grams) powdered sugar

½ cup (95 grams) bittersweet chocolate chips

recipe continues

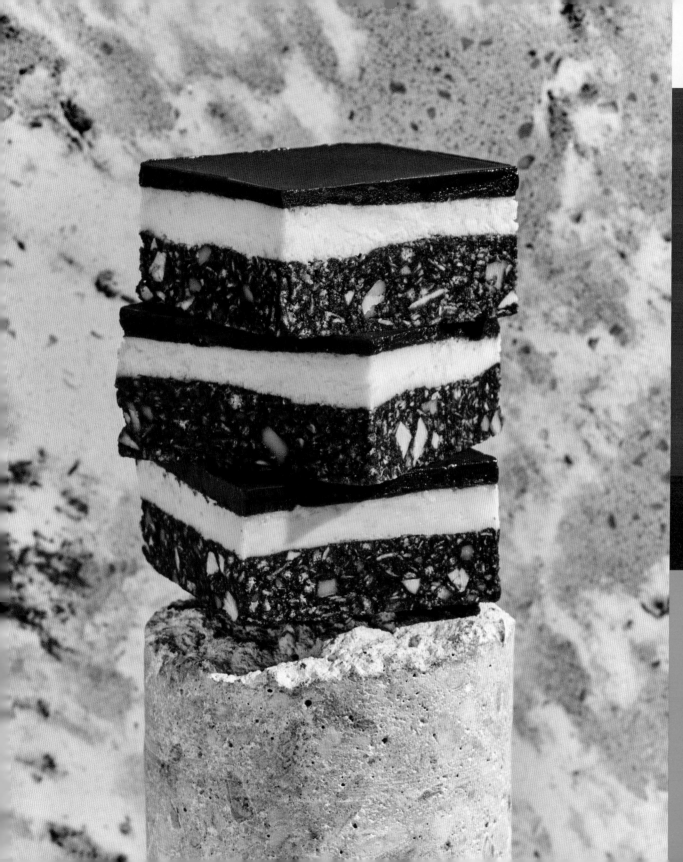

4 **/** Use a rubber spatula to scoop the buttercream onto the chocolate base layer. Use an offset spatula to spread the buttercream evenly. Put the pan back in the fridge for another 15 minutes (30 on a hot day) to let the buttercream set.

5 **/** A few minutes before the buttercream finishes chilling, make the final layer: a bittersweet ganache. In a small saucepan, melt the remaining ¼ cup of unsalted butter over low heat. Turn the heat off and add the chocolate chips to the saucepan. Use a rubber spatula to stir until the chocolate melts and mixes with the butter, 1 to 2 minutes.

6 **/** Pour the ganache over the buttercream layer and spread evenly with the offset spatula. Put the baking pan back in the fridge to cool for another hour and then cut into 16 even squares.

7 **/** Let the bars sit at room temperature for 30 minutes before serving to allow the buttercream to soften. To store the Nanaimo Bars, keep in a labeled airtight container with a lid for up to a week.

SILLY VANILLY WAFERS

MAKES 60 wafers

TIME: 25 minutes

DOSE: 2 mg THC
per wafer

The unassuming vanilla wafer serves as backbone to a number of American desserts, which makes them an ideal edible. Crush them with butter for a quick pie crust, layer them with pudding and bananas for a Southern classic, top them with cream cheese for my Cherry Cheeba Cheesecakes (page 194), or snack on them straight from the pan. Whatever the sweet format, these microdosed wafers make for a silly time.

1 / Center two racks in the oven and preheat the oven to 350°F. Line two sheet pans with parchment paper.

2 / In a medium bowl, use a handheld mixer to cream both butters until light and fluffy, 1 to 2 minutes. Add both sugars, the egg, vanilla extract, milk, and salt, then mix on medium-low speed for another minute.

3 / Sift the flour and baking soda into the bowl, then use a rubber spatula to combine until the flour disappears.

4 / Scoop the batter into a pastry bag and pipe the dough into 30 rounds, each about a tablespoon of batter and the size of a quarter, onto each of the prepared sheet pans, leaving 1½ inches of space between each wafer for spreading. Lightly wet the tip of a finger and tap the tops of the wafers down if they have peaks from piping, then bake the wafers for 12 to 13 minutes, rotating the racks halfway through cooking, until the cookies are golden brown all over. Transfer to a wire rack for cooling.

5 / Enjoy immediately. Store in a labeled airtight container for up to 1 week or freeze for up to a month.

¼ cup (2 ounces) Cannabutter (page 61), room temperature

¼ cup (2 ounces) unsalted butter, room temperature

⅓ cup (40 grams) powdered sugar

¼ cup (50 grams) granulated sugar

1 large egg

1 tablespoon vanilla extract

½ tablespoon whole milk

½ teaspoon kosher salt

1 cup (120 grams) all-purpose flour

¼ teaspoon baking soda

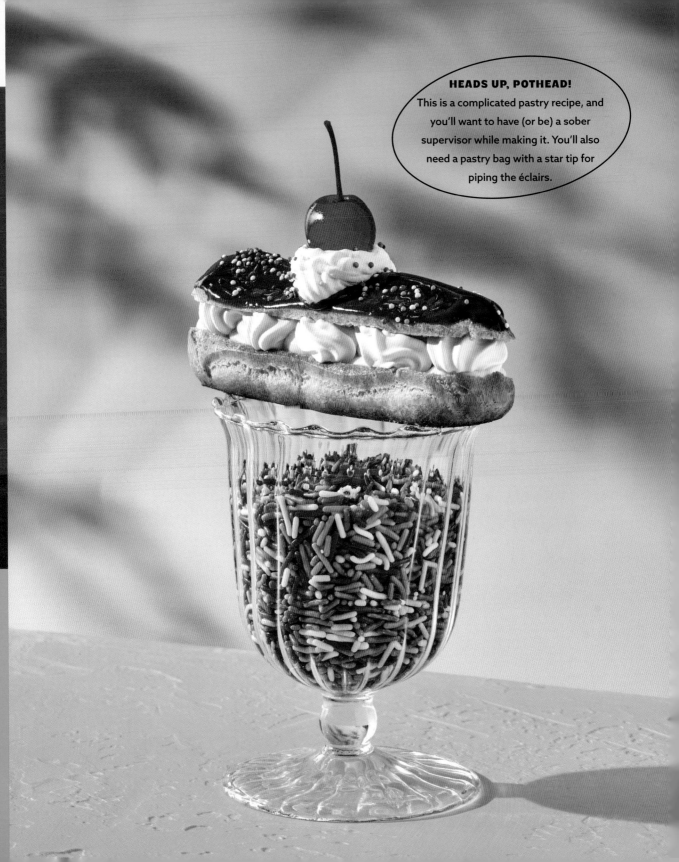

HEADS UP, POTHEAD!
This is a complicated pastry recipe, and you'll want to have (or be) a sober supervisor while making it. You'll also need a pastry bag with a star tip for piping the éclairs.

GO BANANAS SPLIT ÉCLAIR

MAKES 16 éclairs

TIME: 1 hour 45 minutes

DOSE: 6.25 mg THC per éclair

One of my first culinary revelations happened at San Francisco's Ghirardelli Square, where I gobbled down the ultimate banana split, mounded high with whipped cream, chocolate fudge, and cherries. As my palate matured, I often found myself craving a more sophisticated dessert from another Bay Area legend: the chocolate éclair from Tartine Bakery on Eighteenth and Guerrero. To satiate my inner child while still using a refined technique, this recipe combines two San Francisco treats into a celebration of bananas and weed (also a San Francisco treat!).

FOR THE CUSTARD

1 / In a medium bowl, whisk together the egg yolks, mashed banana, sugar, and cornstarch until the sugar and starch completely disappear into the banana-yolk mix, about 30 seconds or ten good whisks.

2 / In a 3-quart saucepan, bring the milk and salt to a simmer over medium heat. Temper the eggs by ladling one-third of the hot milk into the egg mixture while whisking. Then slowly pour the tempered egg mixture back into the saucepan while whisking. Turn the heat down to medium-low and continue to cook, whisking, until large bubbles appear and the whisk leaves an impression when removed from the pudding, about 5 minutes. Remove from the heat, add the butter and vanilla extract, and whisk until the butter fully melts and blends into the pudding. Pour the pudding into a bowl and cover with plastic wrap directly on the pudding to prevent a skin from forming. Let cool to room temperature, then put into the fridge to cool completely for at least an hour.

FOR THE CHOUX PASTRY

3 / Preheat the oven to 420°F. Line a sheet pan with parchment paper.

4 / In a 2-quart saucepan over medium-high heat, bring the water, cannabutter, sugar, and salt to a rolling boil. Turn the heat down to medium, add the flour, and use a wooden spoon to stir vigorously until it

FOR THE CUSTARD

4 large egg yolks

½ cup mashed overripe banana (about 1 large banana)

½ cup (100 grams) granulated sugar

¼ cup (30 grams) cornstarch

1¾ cups whole milk

½ teaspoon kosher salt

2 tablespoons (1 ounce) unsalted butter

1 teaspoon vanilla extract

FOR THE CHOUX PASTRY

½ cup water

¼ cup (2 ounces) Cannabutter (page 61)

½ teaspoon granulated sugar

¼ teaspoon kosher salt

⅔ cup (80 grams) all-purpose flour

2 large eggs, plus more, as needed, depending on the flour

recipe & ingredients continue

comes together into a ball and a thin film forms on the side of the saucepan, 2 to 3 minutes. Plop the dough into a medium bowl, stirring to cool it slightly.

5 / Add 1 egg at a time, stirring until each egg fully blends into the dough before adding the next. The dough should be shiny without being runny and hold its shape without being stiff. Depending on the brand of flour, the dough may require an additional egg if it looks too stodgy and matte.

6 / Using a pastry bag with a star tip attached, pipe the choux pastry dough onto the sheet pan in 1 x 6-inch rectangles, leaving 2 inches in between for spreading. Bake for 10 minutes, then turn the oven temperature down to 375°F and bake another 25 minutes, until the pastry is brown all over. After removing them from the oven, use a toothpick to poke three holes in the bottom of each éclair to allow the steam to release. Let cool on a wire rack, hole-side up, for at least 10 minutes before assembling.

FOR THE GANACHE

7 / Place the chocolate chips in a large bowl big enough to dip the baked éclairs. In a small saucepan, use a rubber spatula to stir together the cream and salt, then cook on low heat to about 200°F, just under a boil. Pour the warmed cream on top of the chocolate and let it sit for 2 to 3 minutes. Using the rubber spatula and starting from the center of the bowl, stir in small circles, working the emulsion from the center out, until the cream fully incorporates into the chocolate, 1 to 2 minutes. Add the butter and stir it fully into the ganache.

TO ASSEMBLE

8 / Slice the cooled éclairs in half horizontally. Use a tablespoon measure to scoop about 3 spoonfuls of banana pudding on the bottom half of a pastry or use a pastry bag to pipe it into the éclairs. Squirt 3 shots of whipped cream on top of the banana pudding. Dip the top of the choux pastry in the chocolate ganache and place on top of the whipped cream. Add one more squirt of whipped cream on top, in the center of the chocolate ganache. Repeat with the remaining pastries. Top each éclair with a cherry and make it rain sprinkles over the entire ensemble.

9 / Eat and go bananas.

FOR THE GANACHE

½ cup (3 ounces) bittersweet chocolate chips

½ cup heavy whipping cream

Pinch of kosher salt

¼ cup (2 ounces) unsalted butter

FOR ASSEMBLY

Canned whipped cream

16 maraschino cherries

⅓ cup sprinkles

FORGET MY BIRTHDAY CAKE

SERVES 16

TIME: 3 hours 15 minutes

DOSE: 15.5 mg THC per piece

The light-as-air burnt almond cake from Dick's Bakery in San Jose made my many six-hour drives from Los Angeles to San Francisco a lot sweeter. One bite of the fluffy white cake, layered with rich custard and sprinkled with salty caramelized almonds, and the miles started to whiz by. Sadly, Dick's went up in smoke in 2016. This recipe pays homage to its California cake and hits at 15 milligrams per slice. I bake it every year on my birthday, which helps me celebrate the day in my preferred fashion: by forgetting about it.

FOR THE CAKE

1 / Preheat the oven to 350°F with two racks in the center. Grease two 9-inch round cake pans with cooking spray, coat with a tablespoon of flour, and set aside.

2 / In a large bowl, sift together the flour, 1 cup (200 grams) of the sugar, the baking powder, and salt.

3 / In a medium bowl, whisk together the milk, vegetable oil, almond extract, and vanilla extract.

4 / In a separate large, non-plastic bowl, use a handheld mixer to beat the egg whites on medium-low speed until they are broken up and frothy, about 20 seconds. Increase the speed to medium-high and continue to beat until the whites turn foamy and opaque, about 30 more seconds. Continue beating while gradually adding the remaining cup (200 grams) of sugar in a slow, steady stream. Once the sugar is all added, increase the speed to high and continue to beat until the eggs get fluffy, quadruple in size, and turn white and shiny, about 5 minutes.

5 / Whisk the liquid ingredients (with the milk and oil) into the dry ingredients until only a few streaks of flour remain, then switch to a rubber spatula and fold in the egg whites, a third at a time, until it comes together in a smooth, light batter, 2 minutes.

FOR THE CAKE

Cooking spray, for greasing the pans

3 cups (360 grams) cake flour, plus 1 tablespoon for coating the pans

2 cups (400 grams) granulated sugar, divided

1 tablespoon baking powder

1½ teaspoons kosher salt

1½ cups whole milk

½ cup OOO Vegetable Oil (page 64)

1 teaspoon almond extract

1 teaspoon vanilla extract

6 large egg whites

recipe & ingredients continue

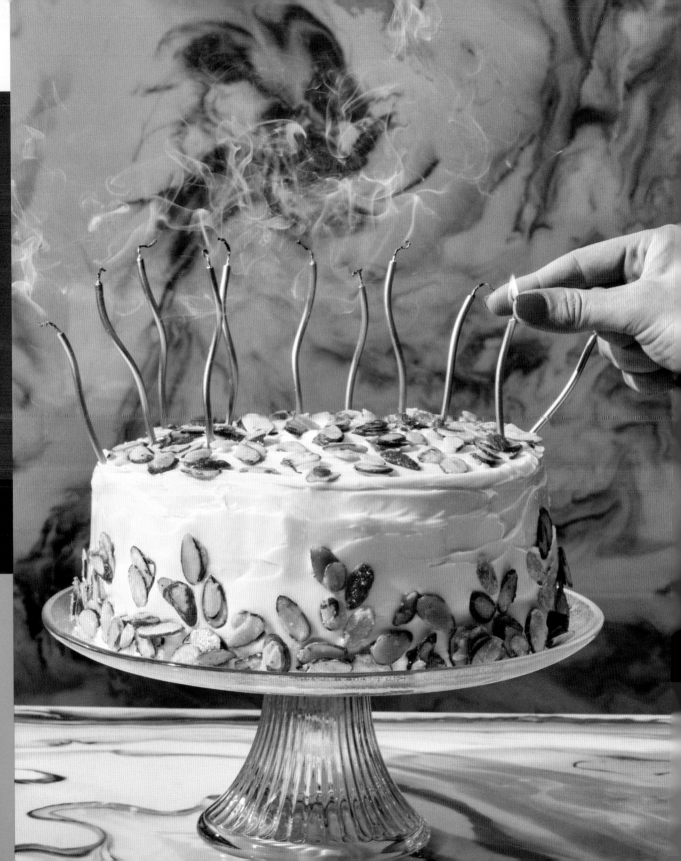

6 / Divide the batter equally between the prepared cake pans. Bake the cakes for 30 to 35 minutes, until the tops are light golden and the outsides just start to pull away from the sides of the pans.

7 / Let cool in the pans on a wire rack for 10 minutes, then transfer to the rack to cool completely, about an hour. While the cakes cool, make the custard.

FOR THE CUSTARD

8 / In a 3-quart saucepan over medium-low heat, bring the milk, cream, and salt to a simmer. In a medium bowl, whisk together the egg yolks, eggs, sugar, and cornstarch. Temper the eggs by whisking constantly while using a ladle to slowly drizzle in half of the hot milk mixture. Slowly pour the now-tempered eggs back into the saucepan of milk while whisking. Continue to cook the milk-egg mixture until several bubbles make big plops, the pudding looks thick and shiny, and the whisk leaves an impression of the wires in the custard, about 10 minutes.

9 / Set a large sieve over a large bowl. Press the custard through the sieve, using the whisk to push it through (this helps ensure a smooth custard). Whisk in the butter until it completely disappears, then whisk in the vanilla and almond extracts. Cover the bowl with plastic wrap, pressing the wrap onto the surface of the custard to prevent the formation of a skin. Refrigerate until cold, about an hour. Use a rubber spatula to fold in the Kewl Whip until the custard looks light and uniform in color.

FOR THE CUSTARD

1½ cups whole milk

1 cup heavy whipping cream

½ teaspoon kosher salt

6 large egg yolks

2 large eggs

2 cups (400 grams) granulated sugar

½ cup (64 grams) cornstarch

¼ cup (2 ounces) unsalted butter, cubed

1 teaspoon vanilla extract

½ teaspoon almond extract

2 cups Kewl Whip (page 198)

HEADS UP, POTHEAD!
In case you don't read the whole recipe, make sure to save the yolks when you separate the eggs for the whites used in the cake, as those are used in the custard.

recipe & ingredients
continue

Space Cakes

How to Eat Weed & Have a Good Time

FOR THE ALMONDS

10 / Line a sheet pan with parchment paper.

11 / Combine the sugar and water in a 12-inch frying pan and set over medium heat until all the crystals melt. Add the sliced almonds and salt and use a rubber spatula to stir constantly until the nuts are lightly toasted and the sugar turns an amber caramel color, about 10 minutes. Turn off the heat and quickly stir in the cinnamon. Transfer the nuts to the prepared sheet pan, spreading them out as much as possible. Let cool before applying to the cake.

12 / Place one cake on a stand and scoop half of the custard on top. Use an offset spatula to spread the custard all over the surface, right up to the edges of the cake. Place the second cake on top of the custard and scoop a quarter of the custard on top, using the offset spatula to spread evenly. Use the last quarter of custard to lightly coat the sides of the cake. Chill the cake in the fridge for at least an hour or until ready to serve. Before serving, break up the candied almonds, sprinkle them all over the top, and press handfuls against the sides of the cake.

13 / Use a large, sharp knife to cut into 16 slices and dish out pieces immediately. It tastes best on the same day, but can be stored under a large, labeled bowl in the fridge for 1 to 2 days. The candied almonds will weep, but think of them as caramel tears.

FOR THE ALMONDS

½ cup (100 grams) granulated sugar

¼ cup water

2 cups (200 grams) sliced almonds

½ teaspoon kosher salt

¼ teaspoon ground cinnamon

COOKIES AND CREAM MINI-CUPCAKES

MAKES 24
cupcakes

TIME: 45 minutes

DOSE: 4 mg THC
per cupcake

I like to take the top off one of these Oreo cupcakes and turn it upside down, sandwiching the frosting in the middle and making the Oreo cupcake into an Oreo cupcake Oreo. This is the kind of meta-munchie you get when you combine the world's most popular cookie with one of the world's most widely grown plants.

FOR THE CUPCAKES

1 / Preheat the oven to 325°F. Place baking cups in a mini muffin pan (or 2 pans, as needed to get a total of 24 cupcakes).

2 / In a food processor, pulse the Oreo cookies for 3 seconds at a time until mostly ground, with just a few chunks remaining, two or three times, then set aside.

3 / In a small bowl, sift together the cake flour, baking powder, salt, and baking soda, and set aside.

4 / In a large bowl, use a rubber spatula to combine the yogurt, vegetable oil, and vanilla extract.

5 / In a medium bowl, use a handheld mixer to beat the egg whites and sugar until they double in volume and become glossy and pale, 2 to 3 minutes.

6 / Add the dry ingredients from the small bowl to the large bowl of yogurt mixture. Fold a few times. Use a rubber spatula to scoop the egg whites into the bowl and fold several more times. When just a few streaks of egg white remain, add the ground Oreos and fold three or four more times to incorporate.

FOR THE CUPCAKES

10 Oreo cookies

1 cup (120 grams) cake flour

½ teaspoon baking powder

½ teaspoon kosher salt

¼ teaspoon baking soda

½ cup plain whole milk yogurt

¼ cup OOO Vegetable Oil (page 64)

1 teaspoon vanilla extract

2 large egg whites

½ cup (100 grams) granulated sugar

recipe & ingredients

continue

7 / Use a tablespoon measure to scoop the batter into the prepared cups, making each three-quarters full. Bake for 8 to 10 minutes; they should bounce back when lightly touched on the top, rather than indenting. Let cool in the pan for 3 to 5 minutes, then transfer to a wire rack to cool completely, 15 to 20 minutes.

FOR THE BUTTERCREAM FROSTING

8 / In a food processor, pulse 10 Oreo cookies in 5-second intervals until finely ground, five or six times. Use a sharp knife to cut the remaining 6 Oreo cookies into quarters to use for garnishing.

9 / In a medium bowl, using a handheld mixer on medium speed, beat the butter, cream cheese, powdered sugar, whipping cream, vanilla extract, and salt until the color lightens and the mixture gets fluffy, 2 to 3 minutes. Turn the speed down to low and add the crushed Oreos, mixing until just swirled through. Scoop the frosting into a piping bag, cut a ½-inch hole in the tip of the piping bag, and pipe about 1½ tablespoons of frosting on top of each mini-cupcake. Place a quarter of an Oreo on top.

10 / Cupcakes taste the best same day, but they can be stored labeled in the fridge for an extra day or two. Let warm up at room temperature for 15 minutes before eating.

FOR THE BUTTERCREAM FROSTING

16 Oreo cookies, divided

½ cup (4 ounces) unsalted butter, room temperature

⅓ cup (3 ounces) cream cheese, room temperature

1¼ cups (150 grams) powdered sugar

2 tablespoons heavy whipping cream

1 teaspoon vanilla extract

¼ teaspoon kosher salt

BLAZED BAKLAVA BLUNTS

MAKES 27 saragli

TIME: 2 hours

DOSE: 3.75 mg THC
per blunt

This version of saragli, or rolled baklava, comes from Greece, where the nut-filled, cinnamon-spiced dessert gets drizzled in lemon-honey syrup. Rolling the pastry simplifies the process, avoids the need to count layers to get the right ratio of phyllo to nuts, and wraps everything up inside the finished treats, making far less mess. Covering them in pistachio crumbles adds extra texture and results in a treat that resembles a kief-crusted blunt.

1 / Preheat the oven to 350°F.

2 / In a 2-quart saucepan on low heat, melt both butters together for 1 minute, then set aside.

3 / In a medium bowl, combine ¾ cup of the pistachios, the almonds, walnuts, ¼ cup of the sugar, the cinnamon, cardamom, and salt. Set aside.

4 / Remove the phyllo from the packaging and carefully unfold the sheets. Have a 9-inch square pan set to the side. Place one sheet of phyllo on a work surface and use a pastry brush to dot it very gently with the butter mixture. Place a second sheet of phyllo on top of the first, lining up the sheets as evenly as possible, and lightly paint the top sheet of phyllo with more butter. Sprinkle a heaping ¼ cup of the spiced nut mixture evenly all over the sheets. With the 9-inch (shorter) side closest to you and starting from there, gently roll the sheet up as tightly as possible. Breaks in the phyllo are inevitable. Place the roll in the pan, seam-side down. Repeat this process with the remaining 16 sheets of phyllo, making 8 more rolls and filling the tray. Use a sharp paring knife to evenly slice all the rolls into thirds, creating 27 baklava blunts. Brush the remaining butter all over the baklava and bake until golden brown, 30 to 35 minutes.

¼ cup (2 ounces) Cannabutter (page 61)

½ cup (4 ounces) unsalted butter

1½ cups (210 grams) finely ground pistachios, divided

¾ cup (115 grams) finely ground almonds

¾ cup (87 grams) finely ground walnuts

½ cup (100 grams) granulated sugar, divided

2 teaspoons ground cinnamon

1 teaspoon ground cardamom

½ teaspoon kosher salt

½ pound phyllo dough (about eighteen 9 x 14-inch sheets) thawed and at room temperature

¾ cup honey

⅓ cup water

1 tablespoon lemon juice (about ½ a lemon)

recipe continues

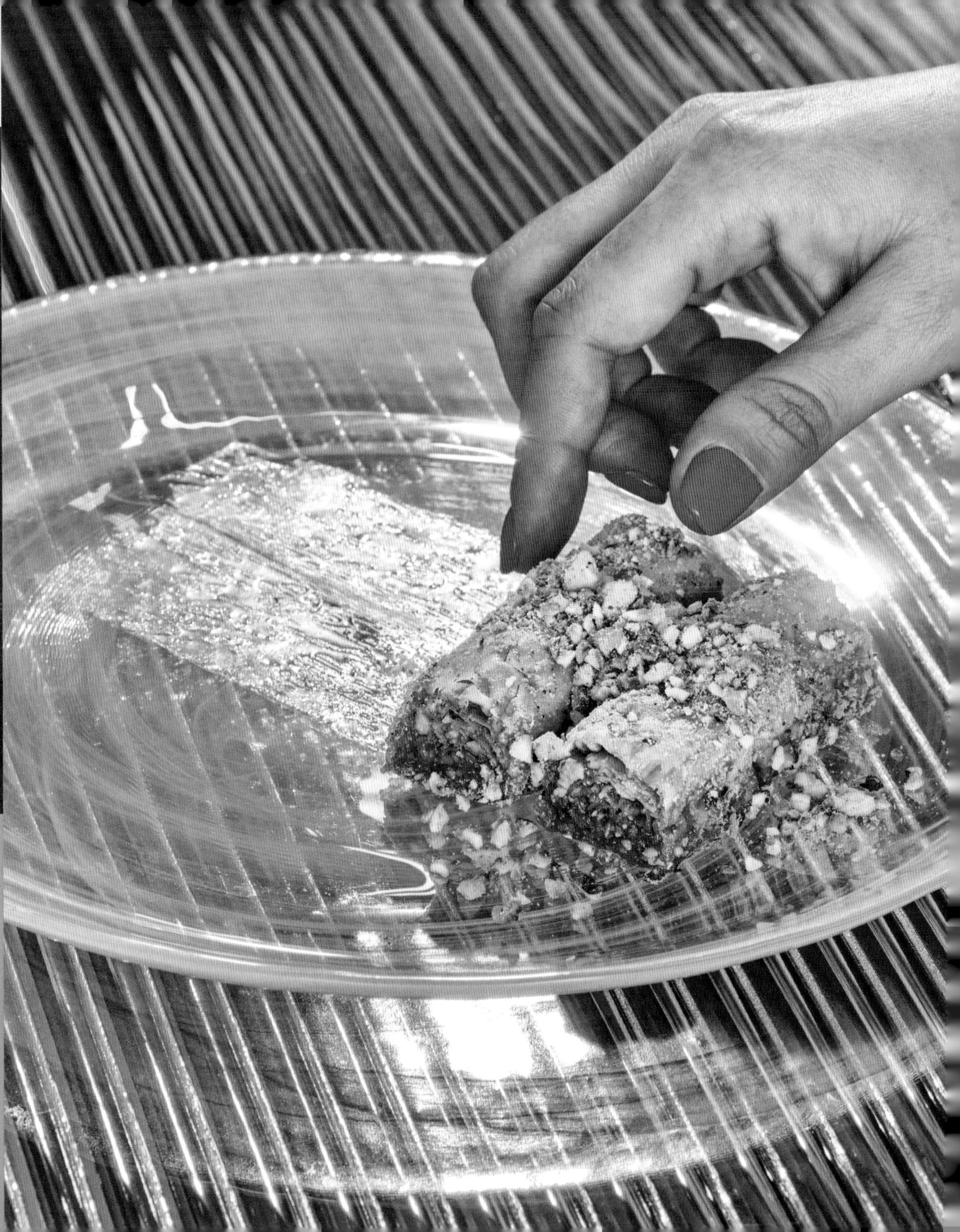

5 / While the baklava bakes, prepare the syrup in the same saucepan used for the butter. Heat the honey, water, and lemon juice and remaining ¼ cup of sugar over medium-low heat until all the sugar dissolves into the honey, about 2 minutes.

6 / When the baklava finishes baking, immediately pour the honey syrup evenly over top. The blunts will sizzle as they absorb the sweet syrup. Let cool for at least 30 minutes. Just before serving, roll each individual baklava in the remaining ¾ cup of pistachio nuts.

7 / Enjoy the same day or store in a labeled airtight container in the refrigerator for up to 1 week.

BERRY WILD POT-TARTS

MAKES 8 tarts

TIME: 4 hours 20 minutes

DOSE: 6.25 mg THC per tart

A stranger on the internet once called me a Pop-Tart pothead, and I took it as a compliment. Pop-Tarts, like potheads, have a lowbrow status to the untrained eye. But Pop-Tarts, and specifically these Pot-Tarts, require skill and technique. The payoff comes from the absurd joy brought by slightly sweetened tart dough filled with a multi-berry paste and glazed in psychedelic frosting.

The key to the filling of this beloved pothead snack boils down to the jam: Straight from the jar, it carries too much moisture, causing the tarts to puff up in the middle. Adding a scoop of cornstarch tightens the jam, resulting in the ideal sticky-thick texture. This recipe also uses pate sucrée, the classic French sweet dough, which requires freezing the dough to prevent it from spreading in the oven. Then comes the fun part: going wild with the frosting colors.

1 / In a stand mixer with the paddle attachment, cream both butters, the granulated sugar, and ½ teaspoon of the salt on medium speed until lightened in color, about 2 minutes. Add the whole egg and beat for another minute. Stop the mixer to scrape down the sides to fully mix the batter, then pour in the milk and vanilla extract and beat on medium speed for another minute to incorporate.

2 / Sift the flour into the bowl of the mixer and mix on low speed until the flour blends into the dough, about a minute, scraping down the sides after 30 seconds. Divide the dough into two pieces and form each roughly into a rectangle. Wrap the rectangles in plastic and chill in the refrigerator until fully cold, at least an hour.

3 / When the dough is chilled, remove from the fridge to soften at room temperature. In a small bowl, microwave the jam for 30 seconds, until just warm. Stir in the cornstarch and set aside to cool completely, about 5 minutes.

2 tablespoons (1 ounce) Cannabutter (page 61), room temperature

½ cup plus 2 tablespoons (5 ounces) unsalted butter, room temperature

½ cup (100 grams) granulated sugar

1 teaspoon kosher salt, divided

1 large egg, plus 1 large egg white

1 tablespoon whole milk

1 teaspoon vanilla extract

3 cups (345 grams) all-purpose flour, plus more for dusting work surface

½ cup mixed berry jam

1 tablespoon cornstarch

1½ cups (180 grams) powdered sugar

1 drop water

2 drops food coloring (1 each of 2 different colors)

recipe continues

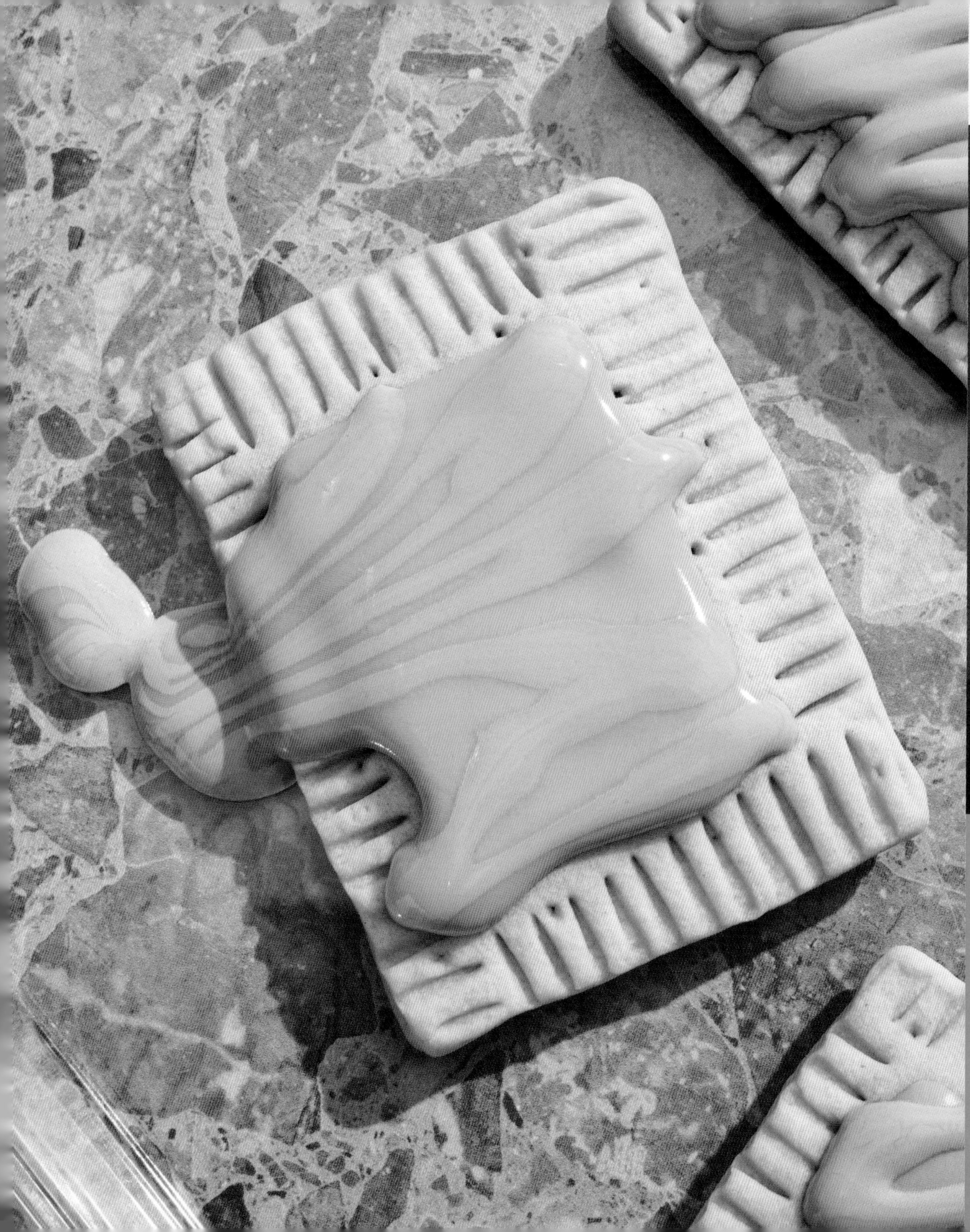

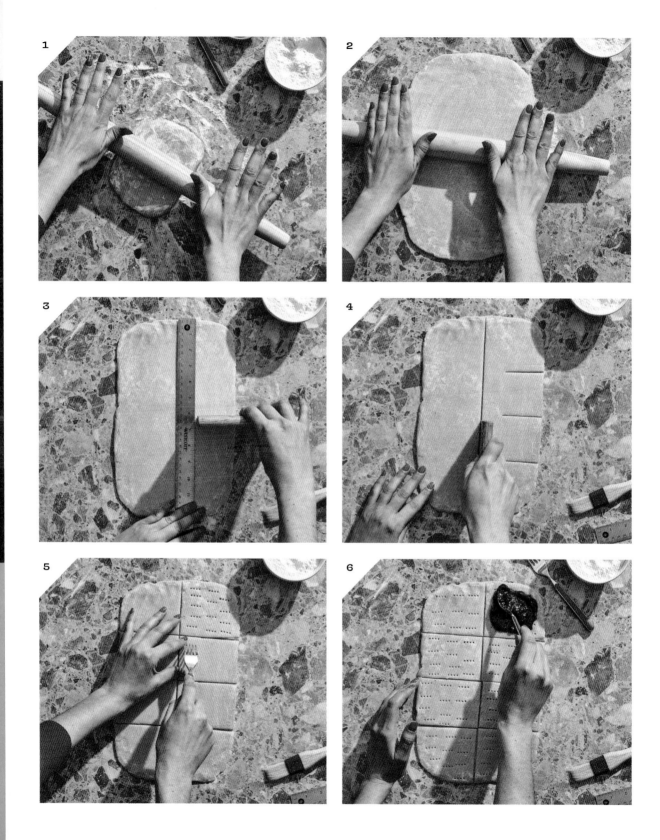

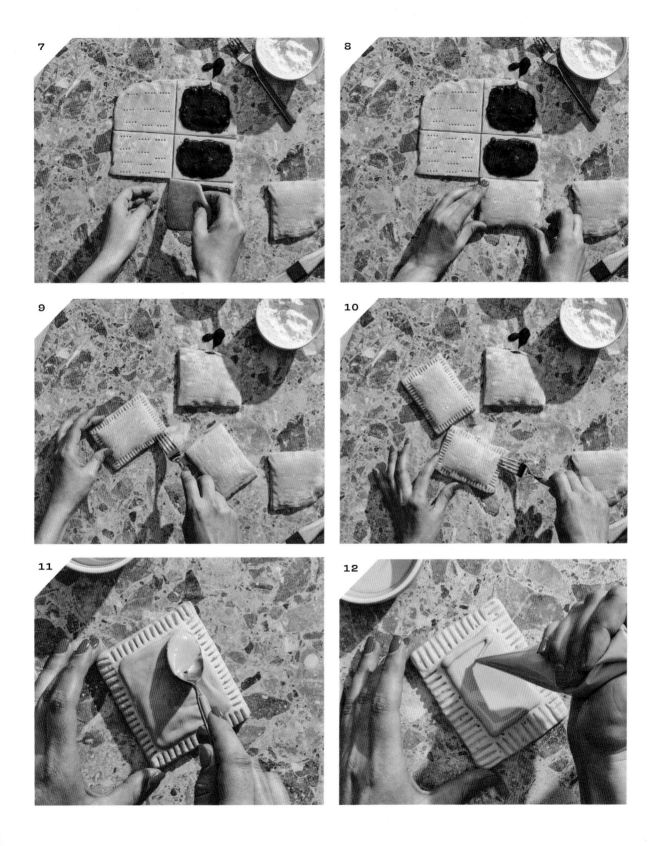

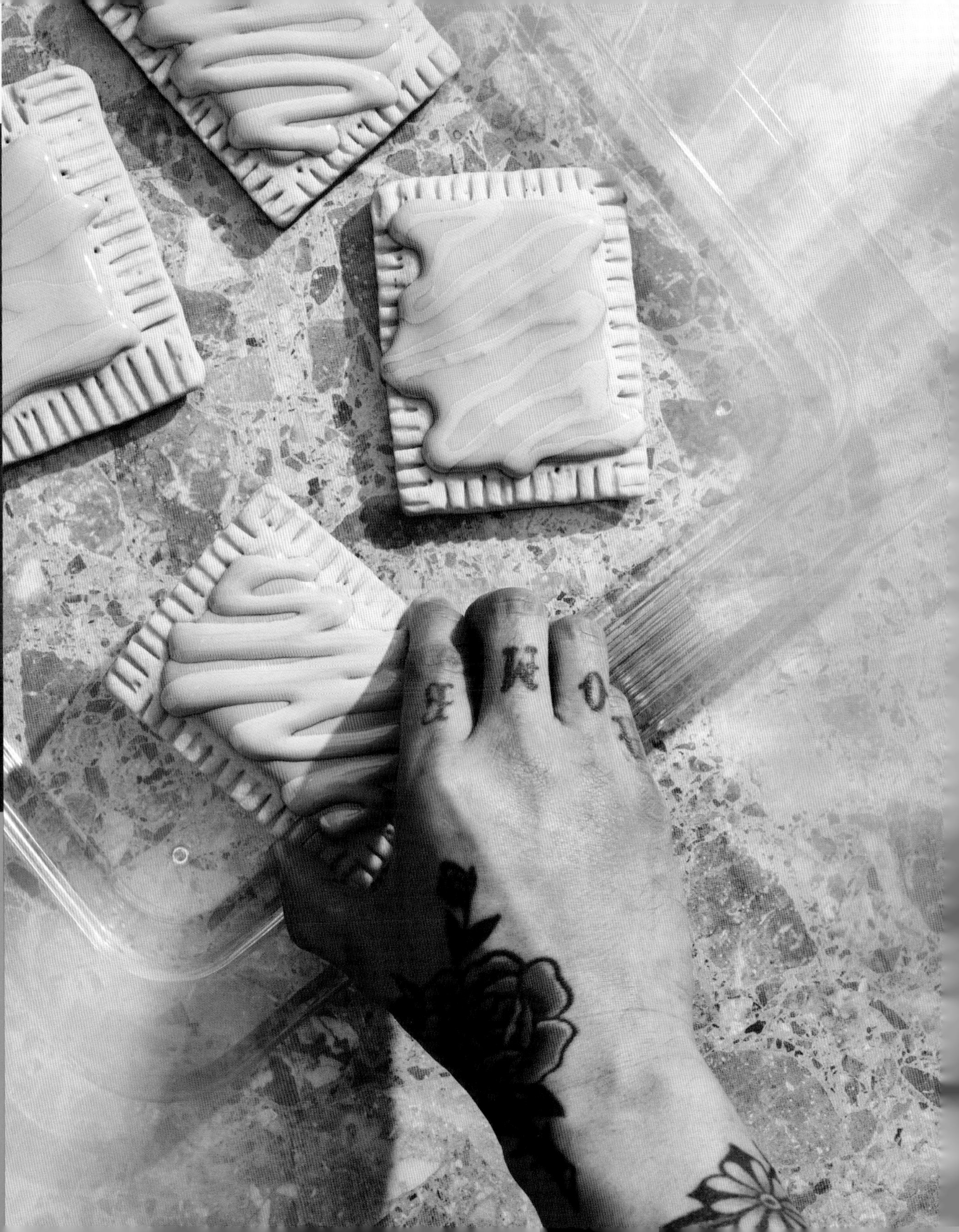

4 / Generously dust a work surface with flour and roll each dough half out into a 7 x 12-inch rectangle measuring ¼ inch thick. Cut each rectangle into 4 strips, lengthwise, so they measure 3 x 7 inches. Cut each strip in half so you end up with 16 rectangles, all 3 x 3½ inches. If the dough gets too soft or misshapen at any time, put it in the fridge and reroll it; you can do this up to three times with any piece of dough.

5 / With a fork, prick the dough all over to allow for steam ventilation. Place 8 of the squares on a parchment-paper-lined sheet pan. Spoon a tablespoon of jam into the center of each of the rectangles on the pan. Spread the filling out in a level layer, leaving a quarter-inch border all the way around for when you seal the tart together. If you notice the dough getting soft, pop it back in the fridge or freezer to firm up before proceeding. Place a jam-less rectangle of dough on top of a jammy rectangle, then press down all around the edges with a fork to crimp and seal them together. Repeat with the remaining rectangles, so you have 8 complete tarts. Place the tarts in the freezer for at least an hour.

6 / Preheat the oven to 350°F.

7 / Bake the tarts, straight from the freezer, for about 25 minutes, until the bottoms turn golden brown but the tops remain pale. Use a spatula to transfer the tarts to a wire rack to cool for 15 to 20 minutes.

8 / Use a handheld mixer on low speed to whisk the egg white until frothy. Continue whisking as you add the powdered sugar ¼ cup at a time. Once all the sugar is added, turn the mixer speed to high and beat until the whites hold stiff peaks, about 5 minutes. Thin the icing out with the drop of water and separate it into two bowls. Add 1 drop of one food coloring to one of the bowls and 1 drop of the other color to the other bowl. Use two separate small spoons to mix each to a consistent color.

9 / Using one of the small spoons, add one of the icings to the top of the cooled tarts, spreading the icing from edge to edge with the back of the spoon. Repeat with the remaining tarts, then let the icing set for 2 minutes. Use the other small spoon to fling or drizzle a splatter of the second icing color on top of the first, à la Jackson Pollock.

10 / The tarts taste best on the first day but stay delicious for up to 3 days when stored in a labeled airtight container.

CHERRY CHEEBA CHEESECAKES

MAKES 48 mini cheesecakes

TIME: 30 minutes

DOSE: 3.5 mg THC per cheesecake

The ancient Greeks baked the first cheesecake as an energy food; athletes ate the honey-sweetened cooked cheese during the original Olympic games. The English took cheesecake a step further, adding eggs to the cheese and nestling it into a pastry base. In classic American fashion, corporations got involved and Kraft swapped the curd for cream cheese. Now the stoners added a special ingredient, and when you dish out these two-bite mini-cheesecakes, guests will say, "I ate the world to find you."

1 / Preheat the oven to 350°F with convection. Line 2 mini muffin pans with baking cups.

2 / Use a food processor to blitz the wafers into small crumbs. Use a heaping teaspoon to evenly divide the crumbs into each cup, then use the back of the teaspoon to press them into the bottom, and set aside.

3 / In a large bowl, use a handheld mixer on medium-low speed to beat the cream cheese, both sugars, lemon zest, vanilla extract, and salt until smooth, about 1 minute. Then add the eggs and egg yolks and continue mixing until just blended, 30 seconds.

4 / Scoop a heaping tablespoon of the batter into each prepared cup of the muffin pan. They should be filled almost to the top. Lightly tap the pan on the countertop a few times or use the back of the spoon to level the tops.

5 / Bake for 13 to 14 minutes, until the cheesecakes puff up slightly but still have a wobble. Let cool on a rack for 10 minutes, then top each cake with a teaspoon of pie filling and a cherry.

6 / Cover with plastic wrap and cool in the refrigerator for several hours before serving. They taste even better the next day but only last for up to 3 days, labeled in the refrigerator.

48 Silly Vanilly Wafers (page 175)

2 cups (16 ounces) cream cheese, room temperature

½ cup (100 grams) granulated sugar

½ cup (100 grams) Stoned Sugar (page 77)

1 tablespoon grated lemon zest (2 large lemons)

1 tablespoon vanilla extract

1 teaspoon kosher salt

2 large eggs

2 large egg yolks

1 (21-ounce) can cherry pie filling

HEADS UP, POTHEAD!
You'll need 48 Silly Vanilly Wafers (page 175) for this recipe, so get a (pot)head start by making those yesterday. Don't worry—that recipe makes 60, so you'll have a few extra to snack on.

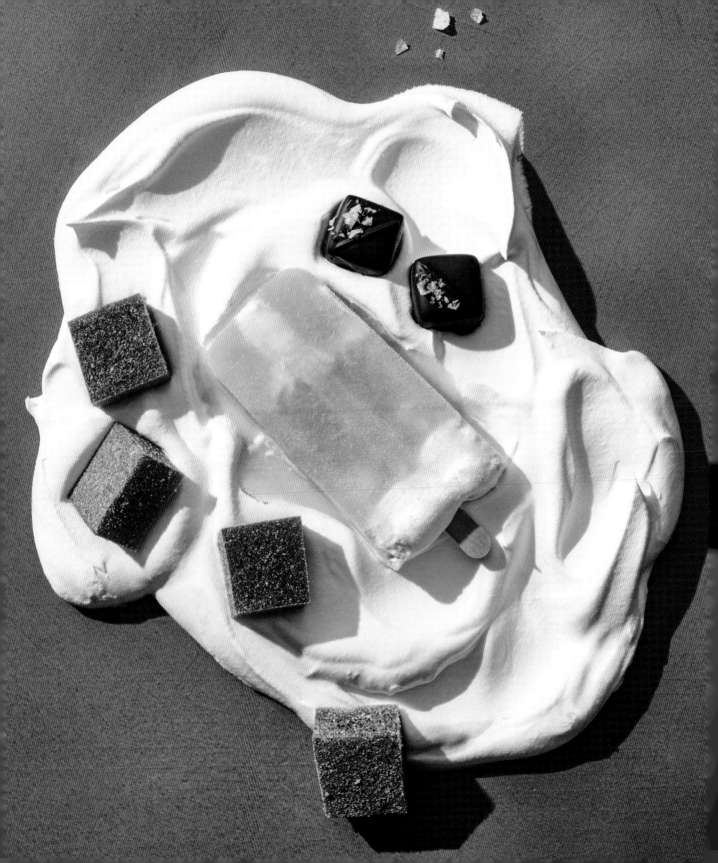

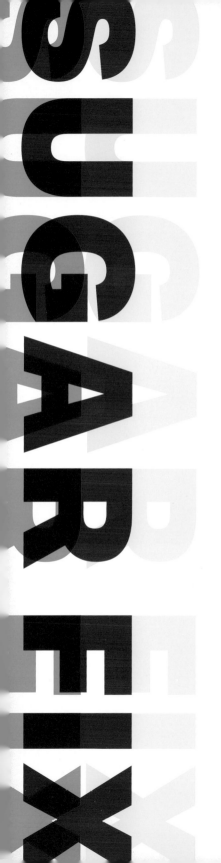

HEADS UP, POTHEAD!
Most of these recipes will require a candy thermometer and a clear head for handling molten sugar.

Cannabis candies delight guests and administer a precise dose. They also have a long shelf life, thanks to all the sugar, so you can get baked without baking and bring out your inner Weedy Wonka with confections that offer a discreet high.

KEWL WHIP

MAKES 5 cups

TIME: 15 minutes,
plus overnight for
chilling (optional)

DOSE: 24 mg THC
per cup

As a '90s kid, I grew up on the Whip: The iconic blue container made an appearance at every birthday party, family reunion, and graduation, topping cakes, accompanying fruit platters, and dolloped on puddings. The joy of opening the freezer to find the quasi–ice cream quickly turned to disappointment the time I found one filled with my mom's one-pot dinner leftovers, instead of the fluffy, lightly sweetened topping. No such sadness exists with Kewl Whip, which is essentially a stabilized whipped cream. The gelatin suspends the shape for hours, and the high lasts just as long.

1 / In a small bowl, whisk together the milk, milk powder, vanilla extract, and salt, then set aside.

2 / In a 2-quart saucepan with a candy thermometer, swirl together the sugar, water, and corn syrup to saturate every grain of sugar. Place over medium heat until the sugar syrup reaches 245°F, 5 to 6 minutes.

3 / In a stand mixer using the whisk attachment on low speed, combine the ice water and gelatin. Leave the gelatin for 5 minutes to bloom, then pour in the sugar syrup. Whisk on high speed, scraping down the sides occasionally, until it turns light white and creamy and appears to have the texture of Marshmallow Fluff, 3 to 4 minutes.

4 / Turn the mixer down to medium-low speed and slowly add the vanilla-milk mixture. Pour in the cream and beat until it makes soft peaks, about 5 minutes.

5 / The pillowy treat tastes delicious immediately but reaches peak Kewl Whip after an overnight chill. Store in a labeled airtight container in the fridge for up to a week or in the freezer for up to 1 month.

¼ cup whole milk

¼ cup non-fat milk powder

2 teaspoons vanilla extract

¼ teaspoon kosher salt

¾ cup Stoned Sugar (page 77)

¼ cup water

2 tablespoons light corn syrup

2 tablespoons ice water

2 teaspoons (7 grams) powdered gelatin

2 cups heavy whipping cream

SERVING SUGGESTION:
This lightly dosed version whips into the diplomat cream for the Forget My Birthday Cake (page 179), but I also like to just eat it with a spoon.

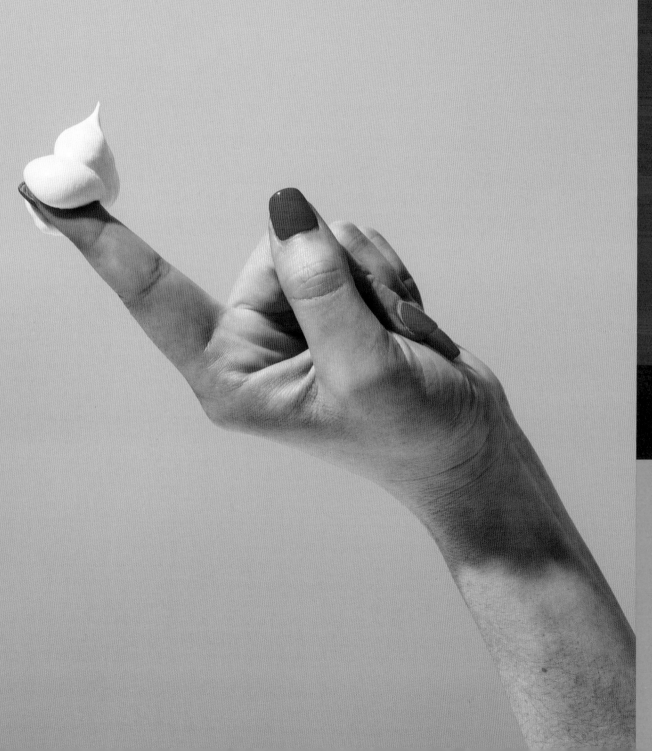

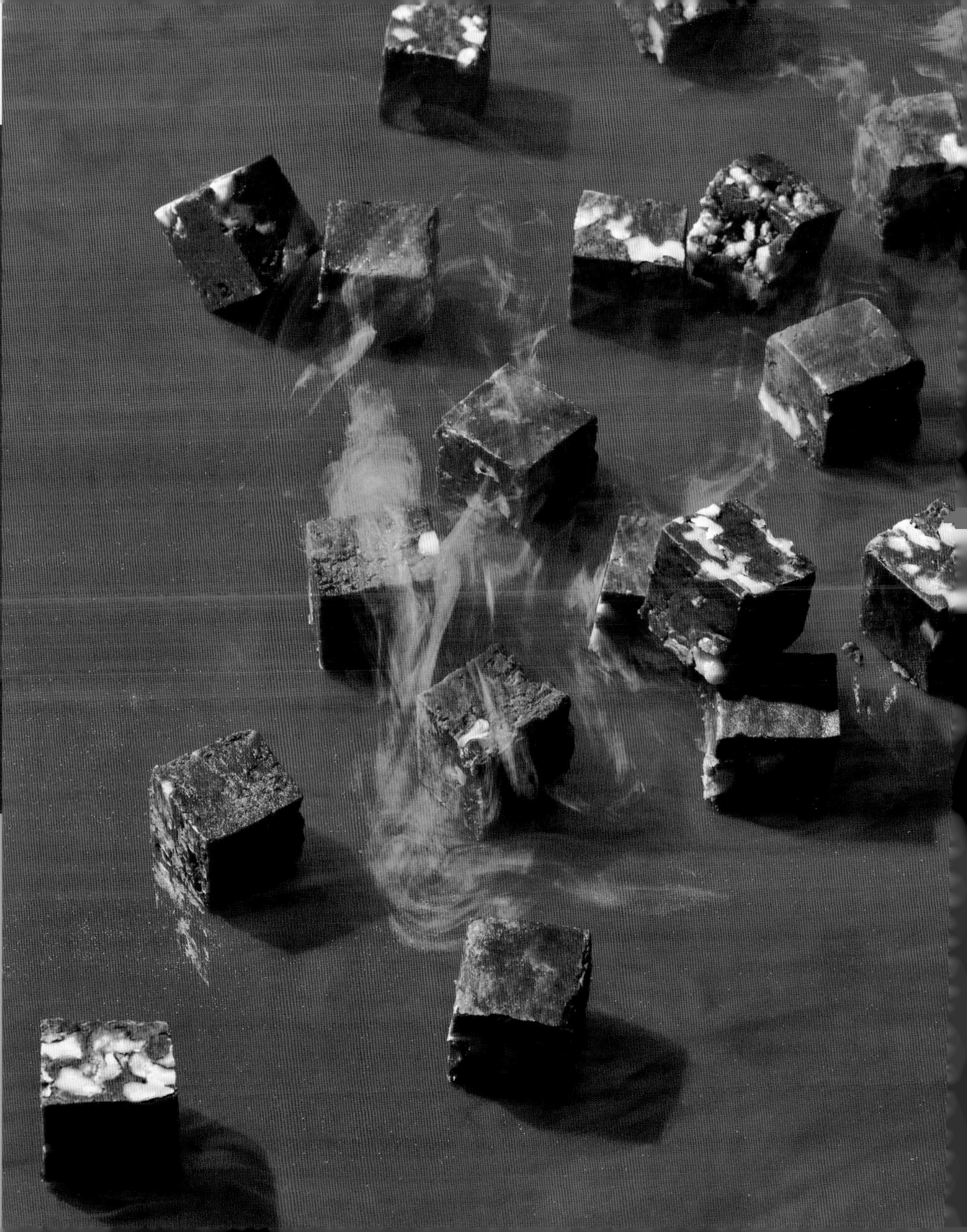

OG FUDGE

MAKES 64 pieces

TIME: 1 hour, plus
1 hour cooling

DOSE: 3 mg THC
per piece

When I was growing up, my dad made a lot of fudge. If I stuck around the kitchen long enough, he would let me scrape the leftover chocolate streaks stuck to the pot straight into my mouth. To keep up with the family demand for his fudge, he relied on the quick trick of using Marshmallow Fluff. This fudge requires more candy-making expertise and time in the kitchen than my dad's shortcut version, but rewards the effort with the complexity of the confection: less sickly sweet than fluff fudge, with a buttery, melt-in-your-mouth consistency. Without the shelf-stable boost, this old-fashioned fudge gets its smooth chocolatey finish from stirring at the right temperature, which slowly, slowly aerates and sets the emulsion as the candy cools.

1 / Preheat the oven to 350°F.

2 / Place the walnuts on a sheet pan and toast for 5 to 6 minutes, until they turn a light golden brown and have a faint nutty aroma. Set aside.

3 / Line an 8-inch square pan with two pieces of parchment paper, going lengthwise and crosswise, with some overhang on the sides for easy removal.

4 / In a 3-quart saucepan set over medium-high heat, use a rubber spatula to stir together the sugar, milk, and honey. Monitor with a thermometer, stirring every minute in the beginning, then constantly as the syrup begins to bubble, until the candy reaches 238°F, about 20 minutes. Stop stirring and immediately remove from the heat and let cool for 5 minutes before adding the chocolate chips, cannabutter, vanilla extract, and salt. Wait to stir until the candy reaches 115°F, about 15 more minutes. The residual heat from the candy will melt the chocolate and butter. Once the temperature cools enough, stir the candy vigorously until the candy goes from a loose chocolate to a thickened fudge that just looks matte, 1 to 2 minutes, then add the nuts, if using. Continue stirring until the nuts get evenly distributed throughout the fudge.

1 cup (120 grams) chopped walnuts or pecans (optional)

2 cups (400 grams) granulated sugar

1¼ cups whole milk

1 tablespoon honey

2 cups (12 ounces) bittersweet chocolate chips

½ cup (4 ounces) Cannabutter (page 61), room temperature

1½ tablespoons vanilla extract

½ teaspoon kosher salt

recipe continues

5 / Use the rubber spatula to plop the fudge into the lined pan, pressing the candy into all the corners and edges of the pan. Let cool completely, about an hour, before cutting into 64 one-inch pieces.

6 / Enjoy immediately. For longer storage of up to 2 weeks in a cool place, keep labeled, whole, and wrapped tightly in parchment, then plastic wrap. Cut off squares as desired.

HEADS UP, POTHEAD!
This recipe requires patience and a strong arm. Stirring the candy before it properly cools makes the fudge grainy, rather than smooth.

PEANUT BUTTER REDEYES

MAKES 40

TIME: 2 hours

DOSE: 2.5 mg THC
per bonbon

Ohio's state candy, the Buckeye, gets its name from a local nut that looks like the eye of a deer; the Redeye gets its name from the bloodshot eye of a pothead. This classic Midwest treat of a peanut butter ball partially submerged in dark chocolate gets its stoner streaks from a strawberry powder iris.

1 / Line a sheet pan with parchment paper. In a large bowl, use a handheld mixer to mix the peanut butter, unsalted butter, and molasses until the molasses completely disappears. Sift the powdered sugar into the bowl, about 1 cup at a time, stirring it until fully incorporated after each addition. Stir in the vanilla extract and salt.

2 / Weigh the dough and divide the total by 40 to see how much each ball should weigh, likely 24 to 25 grams. Weigh out and roll chunks of dough into balls and place them on the prepared sheet pan.

3 / In a food processor, blitz the freeze-dried strawberries into a fine powder, then sift out any remaining chunks. Pour the powder into a small bowl. Dip the top of each peanut butter ball in the powder, then replace on the sheet pan, red eye up. Freeze for at least 30 minutes.

4 / Make a double boiler by filling a 3-quart saucepan with 2 cups of water and placing a medium metal bowl on top. Set the double boiler over low heat. In the bowl, use a rubber spatula to stir together the chocolate chips and coconut oil until they melt, about 5 minutes.

5 / The colder the balls, the easier the dipping, but also the faster the chocolate sets, so work quickly on the next section. Use a toothpick to pierce a peanut butter ball through the red eye, then dip the ball into the chocolate, rolling it so all around the red powder gets covered in chocolate. Turn the toothpick horizontally to wipe the excess chocolate on the side of the bowl and leave the red eye uncovered. Place the dipped ball back on the lined sheet pan. Repeat with the rest of the balls.

6 / Let set in the fridge for 30 minutes before serving. Store in a labeled airtight container in the fridge for up to 2 weeks or freeze in a freezer-safe plastic bag for 2 months.

2 cups Pot Peanut Butter (page 79)

½ cup (4 ounces) unsalted butter, softened

1 tablespoon blackstrap molasses

3 cups (360 grams) powdered sugar

1 teaspoon vanilla extract

½ teaspoon kosher salt

¾ cup (15 grams) freeze-dried strawberries

2 cups (380 grams) semisweet chocolate chips

2 teaspoons coconut oil

PEACH DREAMSICLE

MAKES 10
dreamsicles

TIME: 10 minutes,
plus 4 hours for
freezing

DOSE: 3 mg THC
per pop

A peach pot frozen treat tastes pretty incredible on its own, but piping in creamy Cool Whip cuts the acidity of the fruit and makes these icy treats a dream. While the tincture infuses the frozen fantasy with cannabis, the alcohol in it also keeps the pops soft enough to bite into.

1 / In a blender, purée all the ingredients except the Cool Whip on high speed until completely smooth and lightened in color, about 1 minute. Divide half of the peach purée evenly among the 10 molds.

2 / Use a rubber spatula to scoop the Cool Whip into a pastry bag. Pipe an equal amount of half of the whip into each mold (about 1 tablespoon), then freeze for an hour. Remove from the freezer and pour the remaining peach purée evenly among the molds. Top each popsicle off with the remaining whip and use an offset spatula to level the tops (future bottoms) of the popsicles.

3 / Place the popsicle sticks in the center of the molds and freeze for at least 4 hours before eating.

1 (15-ounce) can sliced peaches in heavy syrup

¼ cup freshly squeezed lime juice (about 2 limes)

¼ cup honey

¼ cup water

½ tablespoon Turnt Tincture (page 70)

Pinch of kosher salt

1 cup Cool Whip

SERVING SUGGESTION:
Amp up the dreams by using Kewl Whip (page 198) in place of Cool Whip for a dose of 5.5 mg THC per pop.

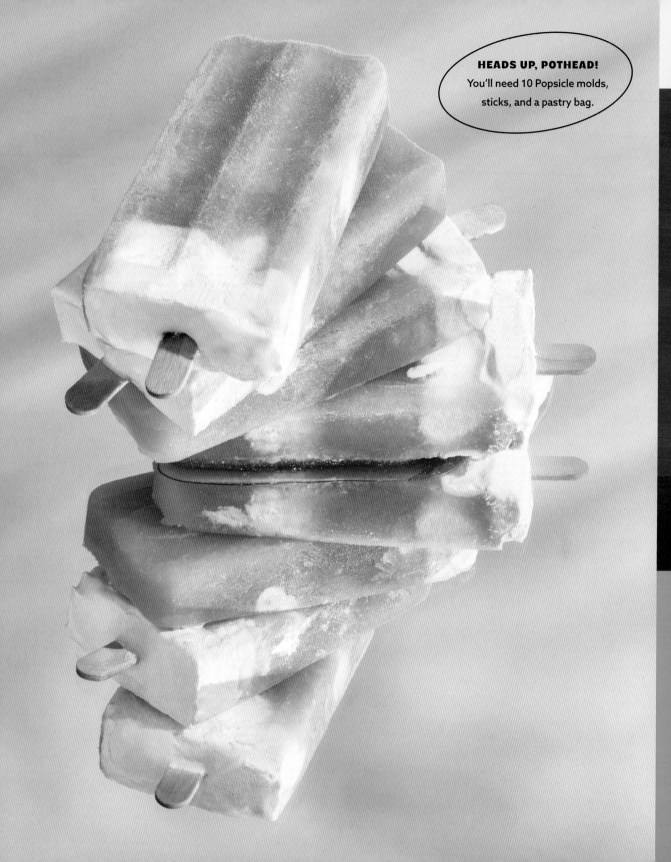

HEADS UP, POTHEAD!
You'll need 10 Popsicle molds,
sticks, and a pastry bag.

PEPPERMINT MIND MELTS

MAKES 16 squares

TIME: 1 hour 30 minutes

DOSE: 6.25 mg THC per square

If a Peppermint Patty and a brownie met at a safety meeting, this mind-melting treat would be their love child. The peppermint takes center stage, making the weed flavor disappear as quickly as the squares do from the pan.

1 / Preheat the oven to 350°F.

2 / Line an 8-inch square metal baking pan with parchment paper.

3 / Make a double boiler by filling a 3-quart saucepan with 2 cups of water and placing a medium metal bowl on top. Set the double boiler over medium-low heat. In the bowl, use a rubber spatula to stir together 1 cup of the chocolate chips with the cannabutter and salt. Remove from the heat, stir in ½ teaspoon of peppermint extract, and set aside to cool. Leave the double boiler set up, as you will need it again later.

4 / With a handheld mixer, beat the eggs on low speed, slowly adding the granulated sugar and scraping down the sides of the bowl, until it turns light yellow and doubles in volume, 3 to 4 minutes. Add the buttery chocolate and blend for another 30 seconds, scraping down the sides of the bowl.

5 / Sift the flour into the bowl and use a rubber spatula to fold until entirely incorporated into the batter. Pour the batter into the prepared pan and use the spatula to spread it evenly. Tap the pan down on the counter a few times to settle the batter. Bake for 15 to 18 minutes—the top will get shiny and the edges will crack. Remove the pan from the oven and let cool completely on a wire rack, about an hour.

6 / In a small bowl, use a handheld mixer to blend 2 tablespoons of the unsalted butter with the powdered sugar, 2 tablespoons of the whipping cream, and the remaining ½ teaspoon of peppermint extract until smooth, about 1 minute.

2 cups (12 ounces) bittersweet chocolate chips, divided

¼ cup (2 ounces) Cannabutter (page 61)

½ teaspoon kosher salt

1 teaspoon peppermint extract, divided

2 large eggs, room temperature

1 cup (200 grams) granulated sugar

½ cup (60 grams) all-purpose flour

¼ cup (2 ounces) unsalted butter, room temperature, divided

1 cup (120 grams) powdered sugar

¼ cup heavy whipping cream, divided

7   /   Use an offset or rubber spatula to spread the frosting from edge to edge, as evenly as possible, over the top of the brownies. Cover with plastic wrap and chill for 15 minutes.

8   /   Simmer the water in the double boiler setup from earlier over low heat. In the bowl, melt the remaining 1 cup of chocolate chips with the remaining 2 tablespoons of cream and the last 2 tablespoons of unsalted butter. Use a rubber spatula to stir the ganache together until the chocolate melts and completely combines with the butter, about 1 minute.

9   /   Remove from the simmering water and let cool for a few minutes, then pour the slightly warm chocolate ganache on top of the peppermint frosting. Use an offset or rubber spatula to spread evenly. Return the pan to the fridge to set for at least 30 minutes, then cut into 16 squares.

10   /   Serve at room temperature or store in a labeled airtight container in the refrigerator for up to a week.

SERVING SUGGESTION:
Dish these out with the Cannabis Chai (page 151) at game night to up the stakes.

STONEY TOFFEE SALTINE BARK

MAKES 40 pieces

TIME: 30 minutes

DOSE: 2.5 mg THC
per square

The key to making a melt-in-your-mouth toffee, rather than a sugar goober that sticks to the crevices of your molars, boils down to the butter-sugar ratio. The butter homogenizes the sugar, but if you add too much, the toffee splits faster than my jeans did the first time I went curling. This toffee recipe prevents the dreaded butter split with maple syrup, salt, and constant whisking as the candy reaches the ideal temperature.

1 / Preheat the oven to 350°F.

2 / Spread the almonds out onto a sheet pan and bake for 3 to 4 minutes, until they turn a light golden brown and have a faint nutty aroma. Transfer to a bowl and set aside.

3 / Line the sheet pan with parchment paper and place the saltines on it in 5 rows of 8 crackers.

4 / In a 3-quart saucepan over medium heat, melt both butters, the sugar, maple syrup, salt, and vanilla extract, whisking the entire time to make sure the candy caramelizes evenly. When the temperature reaches 240°F, in 5 to 6 minutes, pour the toffee evenly over the saltines and use an offset spatula to spread the candy over the crackers. Bake for 10 to 12 minutes, until the toffee turns an amber caramel color.

5 / Use the offset spatula to straighten any crackers that floated out of line, then scatter the chocolate chips on top of the hot toffee and let the chocolate sit for 1 to 2 minutes to melt. Use the offset spatula to spread the melted chocolate from edge to edge. Sprinkle the flaky sea salt on the chocolate and then evenly distribute the toasted almonds. Let cool for 10 to 15 minutes before breaking it into 40 pieces (the saltines help keep the shape).

6 / Enjoy immediately, or store in a labeled airtight container in a cool, dry place for up to a week.

1 cup (120 grams) sliced almonds

40 saltine crackers

¾ cup (6 ounces) unsalted butter

¼ cup (2 ounces) Cannabutter (page 61)

½ cup (100 grams) granulated sugar

½ cup maple syrup

1 teaspoon kosher salt

1 teaspoon vanilla extract

1 cup (6 ounces) bittersweet chocolate chips

Generous pinch of flaky sea salt, such as Maldon, for finishing

CARAMELLOW RICE TREATS

MAKES 16 treats

TIME: 30 minutes

DOSE: 6.25 mg THC

Enough with the super-dosed Trix bars and Cap'n Crunch squares. The marshmallow cereal treat deserves more respect. Rather than switching up the cereal, these bars get a touch of complexity and sophistication from bittersweet caramel blended with the marshmallows. The combination of chewy caramellow with crispy cereal satisfies the stoner craving for textural novelty. Adding weed to the mix just starts the munchie cycle over again, so I always make a virgin second batch to eat after these kick in.

1 / Grease a spatula and an 8-inch square baking pan with butter.

2 / Set a 2-quart saucepan over low heat and warm the cream and salt to a simmer, then turn the heat off.

3 / In a 4½-quart pot over medium heat, use a rubber spatula to stir together the sugar and honey until all of the sugar melts into a syrup. Let the syrup caramelize to a dark amber color (around 300°F) and begin to smoke, 5 to 6 minutes.

4 / Once the caramel reaches the desired temperature and color, turn the heat to low and slowly pour a thin stream of the hot cream into the caramel, while stirring. Add the marshmallows, stirring so the residual heat melts them. Once the marshmallows are melted, add the butters and vanilla extract, stirring until fully blended into the candy. Add the cereal and stir until all the cereal is coated in caramellow.

5 / Pour the cereal mix into the prepared baking pan and use a lightly greased spatula to gently press it evenly into the pan. Let cool on the counter until it reaches room temperature, then cut into 16 squares.

6 / Eat immediately. Store in a labeled airtight container at room temperature for up to 4 days.

Softened unsalted butter, for greasing

¼ cup heavy whipping cream

½ teaspoon kosher salt

½ cup (100 grams) granulated sugar

1 tablespoon honey

26 (170 grams) large marshmallows

¼ cup (2 ounces) Cannabutter (page 61), room temperature

¼ cup (2 ounces) unsalted butter, room temperature

1 teaspoon vanilla extract

6 cups (170 grams) puffed rice cereal, such as Rice Krispies

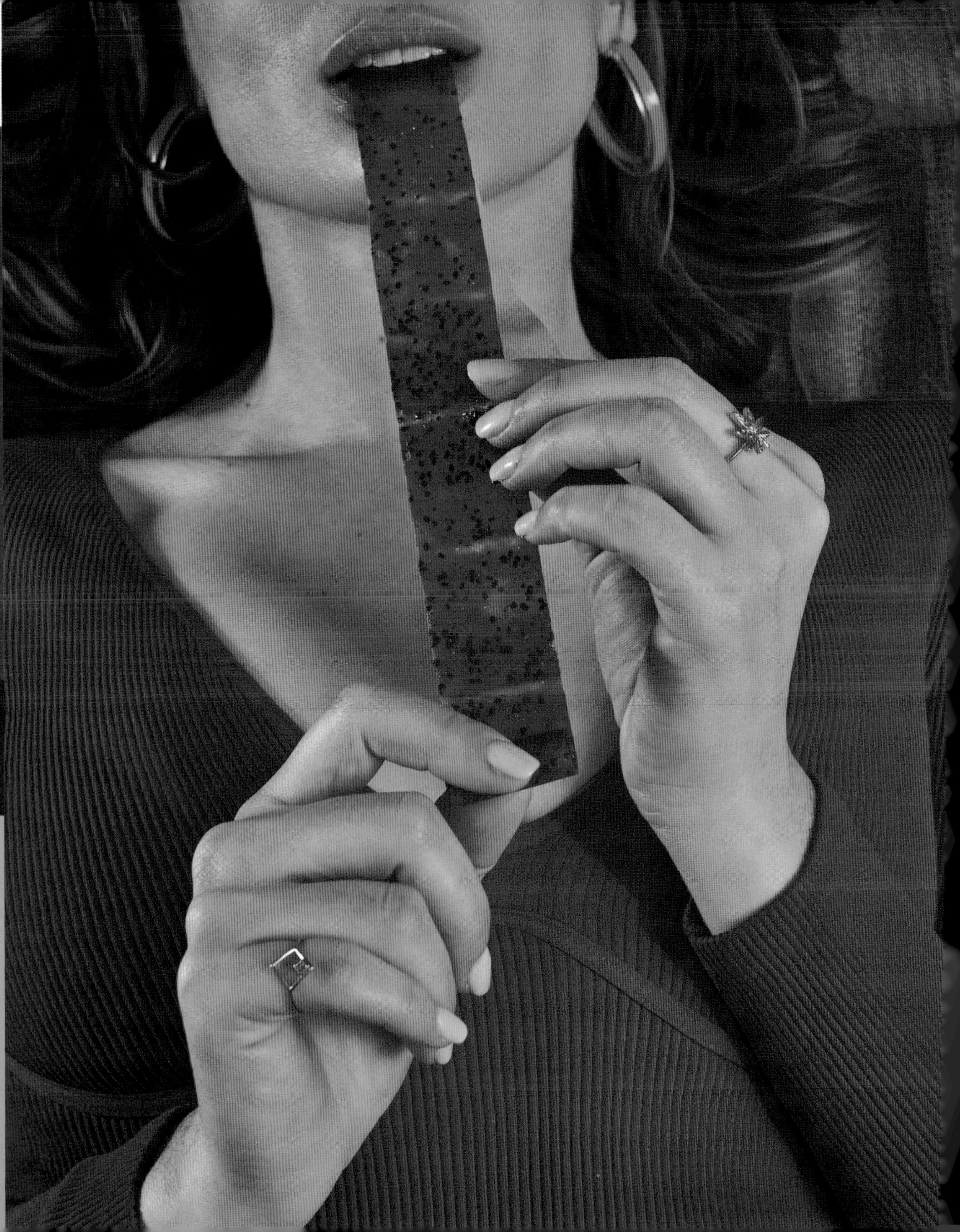

ZOOT BY THE FOOT

MAKES 8 fruit roll-ups

TIME: 6 hours

DOSE: 3 mg THC per roll-up

Roll out your fruit leather and roll up a joint to pass the time, because this recipe requires a little bit of patience while it dehydrates. But once it finishes up, you're rewarded with a milligram of THC in every 6 inches of this kiwi-seed-speckled fruit roll-up.

1 / Preheat the oven to 180°F (you can also use a food dehydrator, if you have it). Line a sheet pan with parchment paper.

2 / At this point, you will separately and simultaneously reduce the fruit purées. In a small sauté pan over medium-low heat, combine the kiwi purée, ½ cup of the sugar, and 1 tablespoon of the lemon juice. In a small saucepan over low heat, combine the strained raspberry purée with the remaining ¼ cup of granulated sugar and 1 tablespoon of lemon juice. Stir both mixtures every few minutes until they thicken and reduce to half the original volume, 35 to 40 minutes. To the kiwi pan, add the coconut oil and give it a vigorous stir to make sure the oil blends with the kiwi. Let both purées cool for 2 to 3 minutes.

3 / Pour the thickened kiwi purée into the center of the prepared sheet pan and use an offset spatula to spread it evenly from edge to edge of the parchment paper. Bake for 45 minutes or until still tacky but slightly congealed together. Use a spoon to drizzle the raspberry purée all over the kiwi, then use the offset spatula to lightly smear it on top of the kiwi without mixing the purées together, to create two layers.

4 / Dehydrate the fruit leather in the oven until it dries out and the top feels sticky but not wet, 4 to 5 hours (depending on the oven). Let cool on a rack for 10 to 15 minutes, then roll the parchment paper up, widthwise. Use a sharp knife to cut the roll into 8 segments, each 1½ inches wide. Store them in a labeled airtight container in a cool, dry place for up to a week, but they are best eaten right away.

1½ cups peeled, puréed kiwi (about 5 medium kiwis)

¾ cup granulated sugar, divided

2 tablespoons freshly squeezed lemon juice (about ½ lemon), divided

¾ cup strained raspberry purée (about 12 ounces raspberries)

1 tablespoon OOO Coconut Oil (page 64)

HEADS UP, POTHEAD!
This recipe relies on the proper quantity of fruit purée, so you will need to make those before starting the recipe. Simply blitz each fruit in a blender or food processor. For the raspberries only, use a mesh strainer to filter the results, then measure the correct volume.

HIGH-WAIIAN PUNCH GUMMIES

MAKES 64 gummies

TIME: 30 minutes, plus 5 hours for setting and 1 to 2 days for curing (optional)

DOSE: 2 mg THC per gummy

These fruity, sour, sweet, and tropically flavored gummies say "Aloha" to a good time. They require a little planning ahead, as the recipe calls for both pectin and gelatin to give bounce to the bites. The fruit pectin slowly sets the gummies with a jammier texture, like in a pâte de fruit, while the gelatin creates springiness, just like it does in Haribo gummy bears.

FOR THE GUMMIES

1 / Line an 8-inch square pan with plastic wrap, pushing the film into the bottom of the pan and letting the edges cover the sides. It will inevitably wrinkle and that's okay, as long as the pan gets covered.

2 / In a small bowl, whisk together ½ cup of the sugar, the gelatin, and pectin.

3 / In a heavy-bottomed 4½-quart pan, combine the five juices and the Turnt Tincture over medium heat and whisk in the bowl of the sugar mixture. Bring the liquid to a boil, then whisk in the remaining 2 cups of sugar.

4 / Use a rubber spatula to stir the liquid constantly until the temperature remains at 222°F on a candy thermometer for at least 3 seconds; this will take 18 to 22 minutes, but part of the candy-making process is the feeling that the sugar will never get there. It will.

5 / Remove the pan from the heat but keep stirring to encourage the bubbles to subside. When they do, pour the mixture into the prepared pan.

FOR THE GUMMIES

2½ cups (500 grams) granulated sugar, divided

½ cup (80 grams) powdered gelatin (like Knox) or ¼ cup for a longer cure

3 tablespoons (30 grams) fruit pectin (like Sure Jell Original)

2 cups unfiltered apple juice

½ cup mango nectar (like Kern's)

½ cup guava nectar (like Kern's)

¼ cup tart cherry juice

¼ cup freshly squeezed lime juice (about 2 limes)

2 tablespoons Turnt Tincture (page 70)

FOR THE COATING

1 cup (200 grams) granulated sugar

2 teaspoons (8 grams) citric acid

recipe continues

HEADS UP, POTHEAD!
Heating the candy to 222°F takes longer than anyone wants it to. Patience is a virtue rewarded with weed gummies.

6 / Let the candy cool on a rack at room temperature (the fridge has too much moisture) until it feels cool to the touch and dry on top, at least 5 to 6 hours or (even better) overnight—in which case, loosely cover with plastic wrap without touching the candy to allow airflow but protect from dust or bugs.

FOR THE COATING

7 / In a medium bowl, whisk together the sugar and citric acid, then set aside.

8 / Use the plastic wrap under the candy to transfer from the pan to a cutting board. Use a sharp, lightly greased knife to cut into 8 rows and 8 columns, making sixty-four 1-inch squares, cleaning the knife occasionally between slices. Toss the gummies, 5 at a time, in the bowl of sour sugar, making sure to fully coat.

9 / Gummies are hygroscopic, meaning they absorb moisture in the air, and sour gummies are especially so, because citric acid is also hygroscopic. You need to either eat the gummies immediately or cure the gummies so they don't weep. To cure (or open-air dry) the gummies and create a skin for longer storage, place on a wire rack in a cool, dry place for 1 to 2 days, then store labeled in a plastic quart container with a lid for up to 2 weeks. Otherwise, enjoy before they get sticky!

MARSHMELLOWS

MAKES 36 marshmallows

TIME: 1 hour 30 minutes

DOSE: 3.5 mg THC per marshmallow

The Egyptians whipped up the first batch of marshmallows using the mallow plant, nuts, and honey, reserving the sweet treat for gods and royalty. Several centuries later, the French stepped in, tossed the mallow plant, and replaced it with a gelatin stabilizer and egg whites for fluffiness. In this recipe, I introduce a new plant for puffiness.

1 / Grease an 8-inch square cake pan with cooking spray, then coat it with ¼ cup of powdered sugar. Lightly grease a knife and offset spatula and set them aside.

2 / In a 2-quart saucepan set over medium heat, gently swirl together (but do not stir) ½ cup of the cold water with the granulated sugar, honey, Turnt Tincture, and salt until all the sugar gets fully hydrated. Use a damp pastry brush to remove any crystals that form on the side of the saucepan. Leave on the heat until it reaches 245°F, about 8 minutes.

3 / In a separate bowl, stir together the remaining ¼ cup of cold water and the gelatin, to bloom the gelatin. Once the sugar reaches 245°F, add the bloomed gelatin.

4 / In a stand mixer with the whisk attachment, beat the egg whites on high speed until they form soft peaks, about 3 minutes. Turn the mixer to low speed and slowly drizzle the hot sugar syrup down the side of the bowl (not directly into the egg whites). The heat from the syrup will cook the egg whites. Once the syrup is added, turn the mixer to high speed for 2 more minutes, then add the vanilla extract. Keep whisking until the marshmallow looks shiny and white and has at least quadrupled in size, 3 to 4 minutes; the marshmallow should be thick enough to hold its shape.

Cooking spray, for greasing

¾ cup (90 grams) powdered sugar, divided

¾ cup cold water, divided

2 cups (400 grams) granulated sugar

¼ cup honey

¼ cup Freezer Turnt Tincture (page 70)

½ teaspoon kosher salt

2 tablespoons (20 grams) powdered gelatin

2 large egg whites

1 tablespoon vanilla extract

recipe continues

5 / Use a rubber spatula to quickly scrape the whipped marshmallow into the prepared pan. Use a lightly greased offset spatula to level the marshmallow out by moving back and forth over the top, as if mowing a lawn. Sprinkle half of the remaining powdered sugar on top and let set at room temperature for at least an hour.

6 / Tip the marshmallow out onto a cutting board and use a sharp, slightly oiled knife to cut it into 6 rows, then again into 6 columns, creating 36 marshmallows. In a large bowl, toss the cut marshmallows with the last ¼ cup of powdered sugar, making sure to coat every edge.

7 / Mellow out immediately or store the marshmallows in a labeled airtight container at room temperature for up to 3 weeks.

HEADS UP, POTHEAD!
This recipe uses the weeklong freezer tincture to minimize the weed flavor in the Marshmellows, which has 50 percent less potency than the standard 15-minute version. Take this into account if you try to substitute (the quick kind will also add some distinctly less-mellow flavors, too).

SERVING SUGGESTIONS:
These spongy sugar clouds shine atop mugs of Pot Cocoa (page 241) and toast into excellent s'mores.

MARIGOLD'S SALTED CARAMELS

MAKES 64
caramels

TIME: 2 hours 30
minutes, plus 5 to 6
hours for caramel
to set

DOSE: 6.25 mg THC
per chocolate

HEADS UP, POTHEAD!
You'll need a chocolate dipping fork
(2- or 3-pronged, though I prefer 2),
a candy thermometer, white cotton
gloves, and 1½-inch paper
candy cups.

My obsession with candy started, like most kids, at the vending machine. While I waited after school for my parents to finish up their teaching jobs when we lived in Alberta, I would scrounge for loonies to buy Mackintosh's Toffee. Making myself comfortable in the library with books on Greek mythology and a stack of Choose Your Own Adventures, I gobbled down the bricks of sticky, chewy caramel. In high school, I continued to feed my sweet tooth by getting a job at See's Candies.

A few years later, when I started cooking with hash, I imitated the candy I knew and loved best, aiming to make infused versions of the top-selling chocolates at See's: Nuts & Chews. As I built my business, my version evolved. I started with caramels wrapped in foil and had exactly one customer. She bought anything I made, as long as it helped her sleep at night. As I refined my caramels, I started dipping them in dark chocolate and sprinkling the tops with sparkly, pyramid-shaped salt. It became my signature treat. This recipe adapts my original recipe to a dry caramel, which gives a superior chew, develops a deeper caramel flavor, and takes less time.

FOR THE CARAMELS

1 / Line a 9-inch square cake pan with 2 pieces of parchment paper, one in each direction, leaving the edges hanging over the sides.

2 / In a small saucepan, combine the cream and fine sea salt. Use a paring knife to split the vanilla bean in half, lengthwise, and scrape the black seeds into the cream. (Save the pod to make vanilla extract.) Place the pan over low heat and use a rubber spatula to stir it every 1 to 2 minutes to keep warm while preparing the sugar.

3 / In a 4½-quart pot over medium-low heat, stir together the sugar and honey, continuing to stir as the sugar melts into a syrup. It will appear to crystalize, but the crystals will melt as the heat rises.

FOR THE CARAMELS

2 cups heavy whipping cream

½ teaspoon fine sea salt

1 vanilla bean

3 cups (600 grams) granulated sugar

2 tablespoons honey

1 cup (8 ounces) Cannabutter (page 61), room temperature and cubed

recipe & ingredients

continue

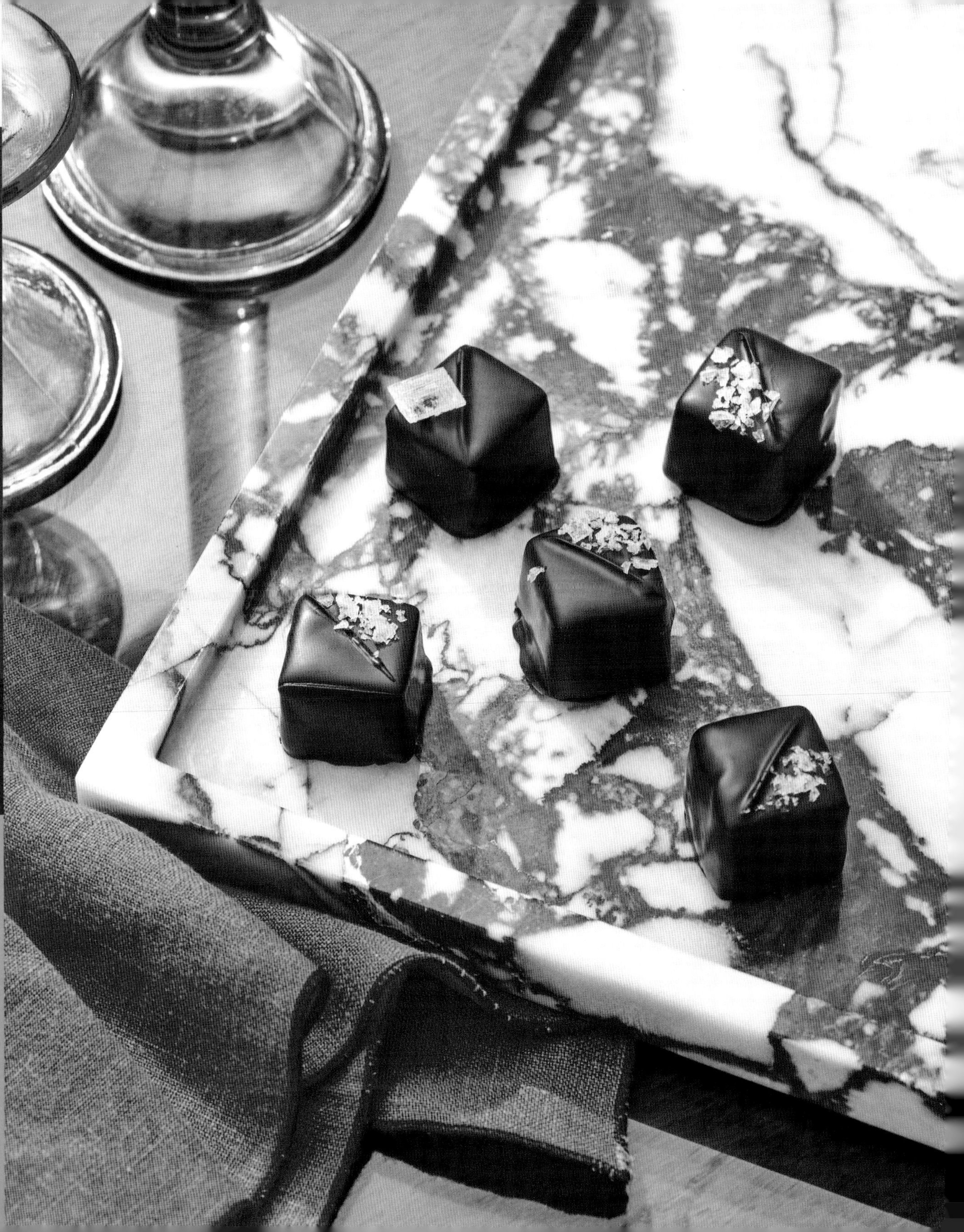

Keep stirring until it turns a dark amber color and begins to give off wisps of smoke, 10 to 12 minutes. Turn the heat to low and carefully pour the heated vanilla cream into the molten sugar in a thin stream, stirring the bubbling caramel to distribute the cream. Once all the cream is added, scrape down the sides of the pot and continue to cook, stirring the caramel constantly. Once the temperature reaches 240°F, add the cannabutter and stir constantly to incorporate. Continue to cook, stirring, until the temperature reaches 256°F to 258°F, depending on the humidity—on humid days, lean toward the higher temperature.

4 / While continuing to stir, remove the caramel from the heat and quickly but carefully pour it into the prepared cake pan. Let the caramel cool, uncovered, at room temperature for several hours or cover with parchment and let cool overnight. The caramel needs to have some firmness, but still indent when pressed with a finger. If the caramel turns out too soft and loses its shape or becomes hard enough to crack a filling, heat it on the stove in the same pot, over medium heat, with ½ cup of water. Stir with the rubber spatula until the caramel melts into the water, then aim for a higher final temperature if it was too soft, or lower if too firm. This can be done only once before the caramel takes on too much bitterness. Once you are satisfied with the cooled caramel, temper the chocolate.

FOR THE CHOCOLATE

2 cups (16 ounces) couverture dark chocolate, divided

¼ cup flaky sea salt, such as Maldon

FOR THE CHOCOLATE

5 / Only temper chocolate on a cool day or in a cool space, ideally below 70°F indoors. Put a spoon in the freezer. Make a double boiler by filling a 3-quart saucepan with 2 cups of water and placing a medium metal bowl on top. Set the double boiler over medium-low heat. In the bowl, melt 1½ cups of the couverture chocolate in the bowl until completely smooth and at the temperature recommended by that specific brand of chocolate in their tempering instructions (usually around 115°F). Remove from the heat and wipe the bottom of the bowl with a kitchen towel. Add the remaining ½ cup of "seed" chocolate, which trains the crystals in the melted chocolate to emulsify. Stir constantly as the seed chocolate melts into the melted chocolate. Monitor the temperature as it melts until the temperature reaches 90°F. At that point, remove any remaining unmelted seed chocolate and put it aside in a separate medium bowl; it will be used later. Keep stirring the melted chocolate until it reaches 88.7°F. At this point the chocolate is in temper. Wipe the bottom of the bowl with the towel again and then test the temper: Dip the frozen spoon into the chocolate and remove it.

recipe continues

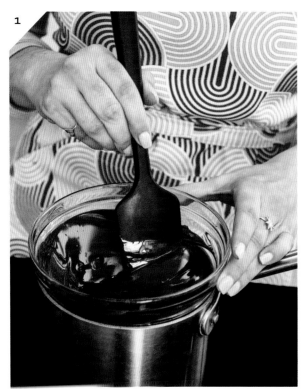

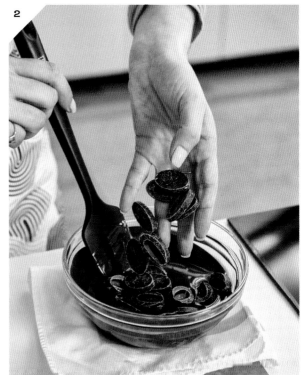

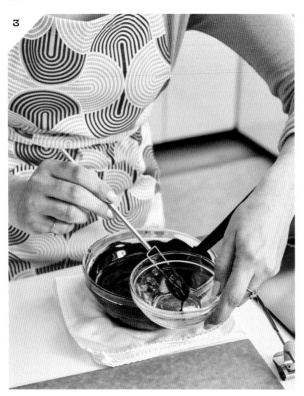

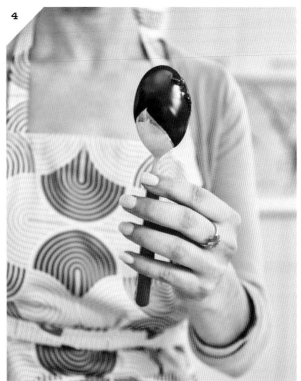

5

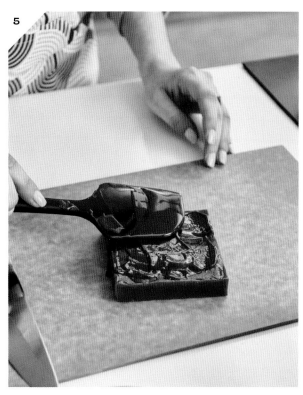

6

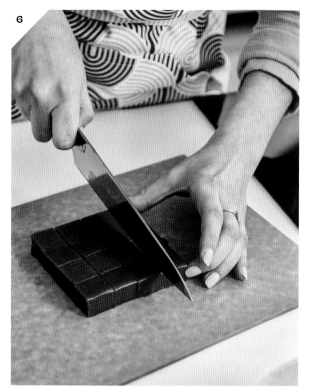

7

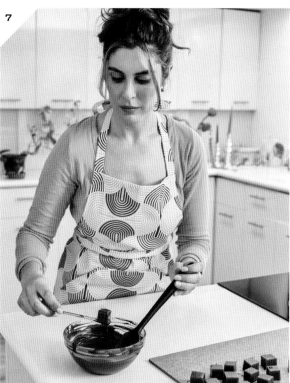

8

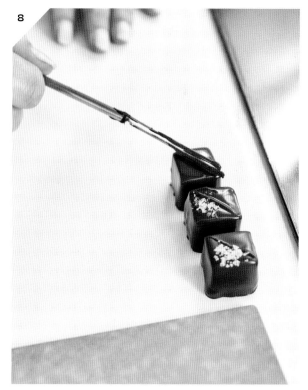

Properly tempered chocolate will be reflective, shiny, and crack when broken off the spoon with a fingernail, rather than appearing matte and smudging when touched. If the chocolate doesn't look right, use the same chocolate and begin the tempering process again.

6 / Pour 2 tablespoons of the tempered chocolate on top of the caramel and use an offset spatula to spread it. This will form the foot (bottom) of the candy, helping it slip more easily off the fork when dipping than the sticky caramel would. Let the chocolate set—which should take just 1 to 2 minutes when properly tempered—then flip the caramel pan over onto a cutting board, chocolate-side down. Use a sharp chef's knife and a ruler to cut the caramel slab into quarters. Put three quarters back in the pan and work with just one quarter at a time so the caramels keep their shape during dipping. Cut the quarter-slab into 16 even pieces by making 3 evenly spaced cuts in each direction. Continue to the dipping stage and finish this quarter before returning to cut the other quarters.

7 / Lay a piece of parchment paper over a work surface. Use a pronged chocolate dipping fork to lift a square of caramel, chocolate-side down. Coat the caramel square in the tempered chocolate by making a J motion with the fork through the remaining chocolate. Tap it on the edge of the bowl, scraping any excess chocolate from the bottom into the bowl and using the motion to nudge the candy closer to the tip. Put the tip of the fork on the parchment, holding the opposite end of the fork up at about a 30-degree angle, and wiggle the chocolate down the slope onto the parchment paper. If the chocolate sticks, use a paring knife to scoot it off. Use one edge of the dipping fork to create a diagonal line on the top of the chocolate by lightly touching a corner on the top with one prong and dragging the prong to the opposite corner. Sprinkle one of the corners on either side of the diagonal line with the flaky salt. Repeat with the remaining pieces in that quarter slab. When the chocolate starts to set in the bowl, transfer any pieces of hardened chocolate to the bowl with the removed seed chocolate. Set the bowl of hard chocolate over the double boiler and melt until smooth and 115°F. Remove from the double boiler, wipe the bottom of the bowl, and allow it to cool to 90°F, then stir it into the bowl of tempered chocolate until fully blended, 1 to 2 minutes.

8 / When the first quarter-slab of chocolates is complete, repeat the cutting and dipping process with the remaining 3 slabs. Let the enrobed chocolates set for 10 minutes in a cool place, then use the cotton gloves (to avoid fingerprints) to place them in 1½-inch paper candy cups.

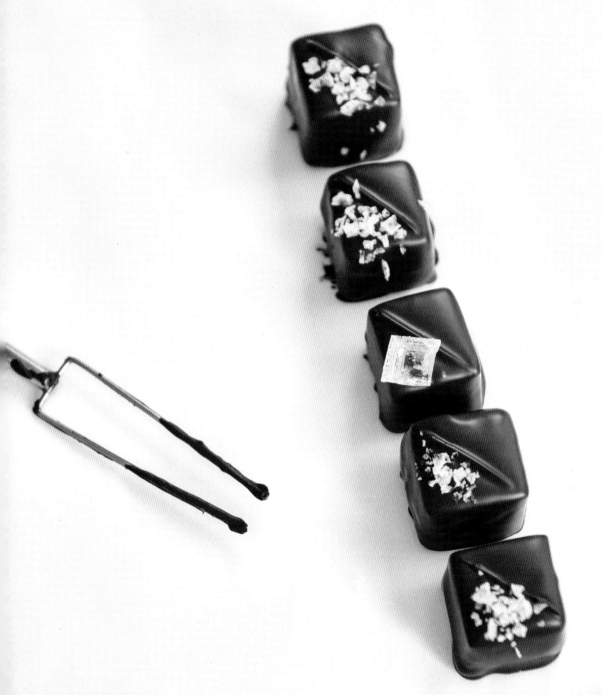

9 / Package the chocolates in boxes of 4, tie a ribbon around the box, and add a note with the dose per chocolate. Store in a cool place (not the refrigerator) for up to a year.

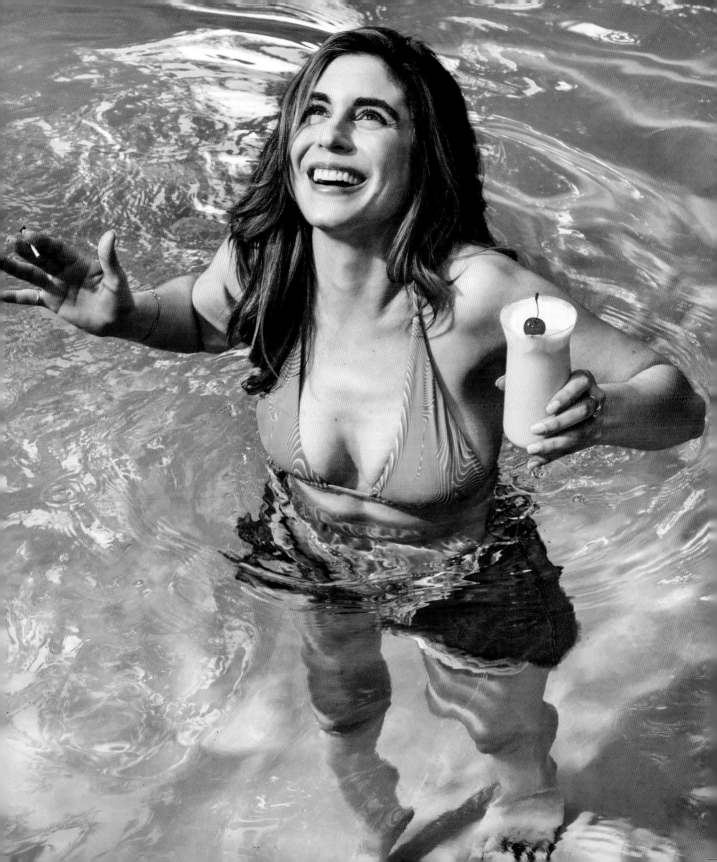

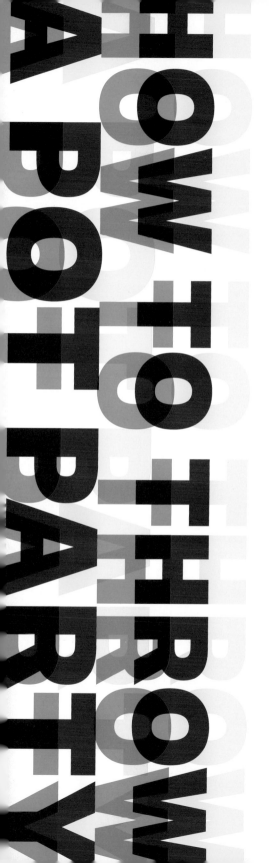

HOW TO THROW A POT PARTY

Real estate agents say "location, location, location" and edible makers say "duration, duration, duration." Edibles last longer than smoking, so throwing a party requires skill and careful planning to ensure the climax of everyone's highs hits a few hours before they head home.

Hosting an infused party takes on a level of responsibility for the guests' experience. Get to know everyone's tolerance before planning the meal by having guests tell you about their experience with edibles when they RSVP. On the invitation, ask guests how many times they've eaten weed and if they know how many milligrams they prefer. If it's their inaugural edible voyage, serve guests a maximum of 2 milligrams THC throughout the meal and send them home with a goody bag if they want more of a high. Sometimes first-timers eat edibles and don't get high, but better safe than sorry.

A thoughtfully infused menu gives guests options to tap out when necessary or ramp it up with added options. Spark appetites by kicking off the party with dosed appetizers and ice-breaking drinks, but keep entrées sans weed. By the time the munchies hit, the uninfused entrées wow the crowd and allow everyone to eat with abandon. For heavier hitters, jazz up the spread with dosed sauces and other infusions on the side. Depending on the information gathered in RSVPs, either offer a lightly laced dessert or send people home with party favors to remember the evening—or to help forget it. At the end, make sure all guests have safe, sober rides or taxis taking everybody home.

SUGGESTED MENUS

Pool Party

Celebrate the summer and soak up the sun with a weed-infused bash by the pool. It turns out there's no need to wait an hour after eating before swimming, so you can paddle around the pool while you wait for your edibles to really get you floating.

MAKE A SPLASHY ENTRANCE: Blend up a batch of **Pot-A-Coladas** (page 158) for new arrivals to sip on.

TAKE A DIP: Set up a table with a bowl full of **Ganja Guacamole** (page 113) and a plate of **Toker Taquitos** (page 82) doused in **Grass Is Greener Salsa Verde** (page 112) and dolloped in crema.

WORK SMARTER, NOT HARDER: In true stoner fashion, the best move here is to order pies from the best local pizza spot and serve them with sides of **Revved-Up Ranch** (page 123) and **Oregano Marinara** (page 118).

FLOAT AWAY: During golden hour, pass out **Peach Dreamsicles** (page 204) to cool off as the sun sets.

Bent BBQ

Two great American pastimes come together when you get stoned and grill meat. Fire up the BBQ and invite the crew over for a backyard smoke-fest.

LIGHT UP: Toast to toasting the gang with **Bong Island Iced Tea** (page 154) and open a bag of chips for the **Queso Extra Fundido** (page 120).

SMOKE 'EM IF YOU GOT 'EM: Slather baby back ribs with **BBQROFL Sauce** (page 119) and tell the guests to lick their fingers.

GET YOUR GREENS: To counteract the meat sweats, serve some roughage in the form of **Devil's Lettuce Cups** (page 92) and a potato salad.

PUT OUT THE FIRE: Pull **Cherry Cheeba Cheesecakes** (page 194) from the fridge for a microdosed finale.

Cannabis Campout

The Thai word for stoners translates to "the green people," because cannabis connects us to plants. Reconnect with nature on a higher level on a weed-infused camping trip. Wake and bake, then maintain the high throughout the day and into the night to help fall asleep under the stars.

BREAKFAST: Brew a strong cup of coffee in a percolator, sprinkle the **Treehugger Granola** (page 134) over a bowl of yogurt, and top it with fresh berries.

SNACK: Pack **Bliss Balls** (page 136) for a hike in the woods.

DINNER: Back at camp, light the fire and skewer some hot dogs on a stick to char in the flames and sandwich inside a brioche bun. Squeeze ketchup and mustard on top, then add a little extra heat from a spoonful of **Cosmic Chili Crisp** (page 124). For a fancier feast, throw a grill over the hot coals to sear juicy rib-eye steaks and coal-baked potatoes, then serve them with **Peter Piper's Peperonata** (page 116).

DESSERT: Before extinguishing the fire, roast **Marshmellows** (page 215) and boil water to whisk up mugs of **Pot Cocoa Mix** (page 241). Topping the cocoa with toasted Marshmellows is optional.

Baked Brunch

The magic time between breakfast and lunch holds a sacred place for stoners because it unifies two top-tier meals into one long feast. This buffet of late-morning bangers will keep the worries of the day far, far away.

WAKE-UP CALL: Kick off brunch with a little pick-me-up in the form of **Chilled-Out Almond Mochas** (page 150) and **Bluest Blueberry Muffins** (page 162) for guests to snack on.
PRO TIP: Have the infused **Faded Sundae Fudge Sauce** (page 234) and a non-infused sauce ready, so guests can decide their own peak.

SECOND SESSION: Move into more savory territory with **Bloody Mary Janes** (page 157) and **Hash Puppies** (page 91) with a selection of non-infused dipping sauces.

MUNCHIE MADNESS: At this point, the brunch should be sufficiently stoned. Bring on the bagels, cream cheese, lox, capers, and red onions. Add a platter of fruit on the side, and, if anyone requests more weed, a bowl of **Kewl Whip** (page 198) for dipping.

Pothead Picnic

Being on grass tastes better while sitting in grass, so pack a picnic basket of delicately dosed edibles and a bowl for an afternoon of al fresco dining.

SNACK PLATTER: Lay your blanket or tablecloth with **Cracked-Up Crackers** (page 135) and vegetable crudité with **Hemp Hummus** (page 122).

LUNCH: Pull out the paper cups and pour lemonade while passing around **Chicken Pot Potpies** (page 86) and a big bowl of green salad tossed in vinaigrette dressing.

DESSERT: Finish the afternoon on a sweet note with **Lil' Nessa's Snack Cake** (page 171).

Movie Night

Who said couch lock was a bad thing? Put on pajamas, grab a cozy blanket, queue up a binge-worthy show or a fantastic trilogy, and invite over the buds. With a lineup of infused snacks and a pillowy couch, this movie night will most likely turn into a slumber party.

SNACK ATTACK: Clear off the coffee table between the couch and the TV to make room for the food. In a large bowl, pour the **Party Crunch Mix** (page 133) and set it in the center of the table flanked by **Hot Honey Firecrackers** (page 139) and **Chili Ranch Tortilla Chips** (page 130).

INTERMISSION: Midway through, stop to broil the **Thrice-Baked Couch Potatoes** (page 84), microwave a bag of popcorn, and blend up **Cereal Chiller Milkshakes** (page 152).

NIGHTCAP: Say sweet dreams with a **Cannabis Chai** (page 151) and **Berry Wild Pot-Tarts** (page 188).

Stoner Soirée

It feels good to get dressed up and even better to get stoned, so throw a fancy, faded fête. Impress guests with an elevated evening that takes them from infused amuse-bouche to dank goody bags.

WELCOME DRINK: Greet guests with **The Grape Beyond Fizz** (page 148) and olives or mixed nuts to nibble.

APPETIZERS: When everyone has a drink in hand, pass around the **Green Gougères** (page 94) and cantaloupe slices wrapped in prosciutto.

ENTRÉE: Once the buzz starts to hit, invite the party to take their seats for the main course of eggplant Parmesan—with a side of **Oregano Marinara** (page 118) for the seasoned stoners.

DESSERT: Serve **Rosemary-Jane Biscotti** (page 238) and vin santo.

PARTY FAVORS: Send everyone off with a little bottle of **Lit Limoncello** (page 237) and baggie of **Love Thyself Lavender Bath Salts** (page 242).

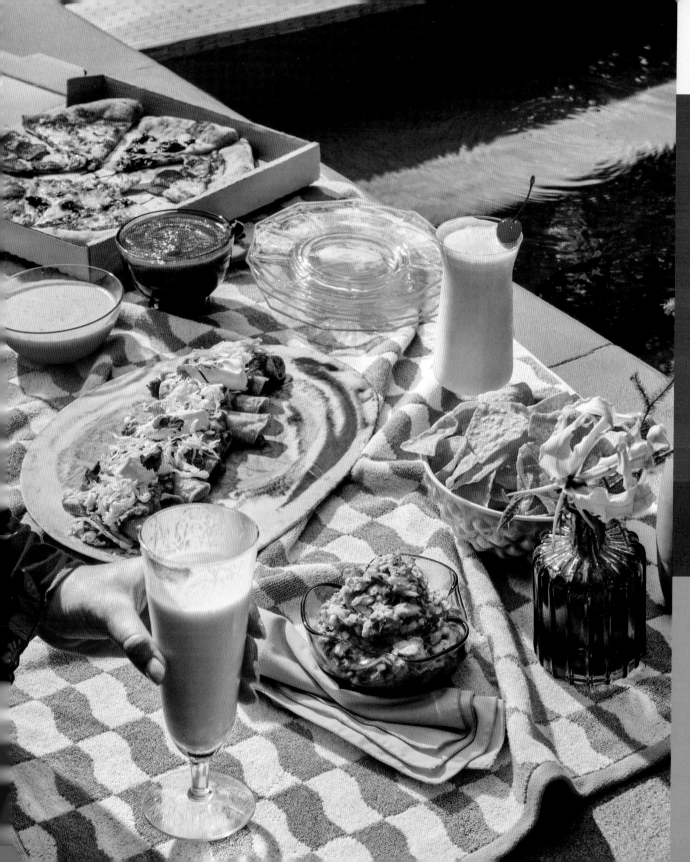

How to Throw a Pot Party

How to Eat Weed & Have a Good Time

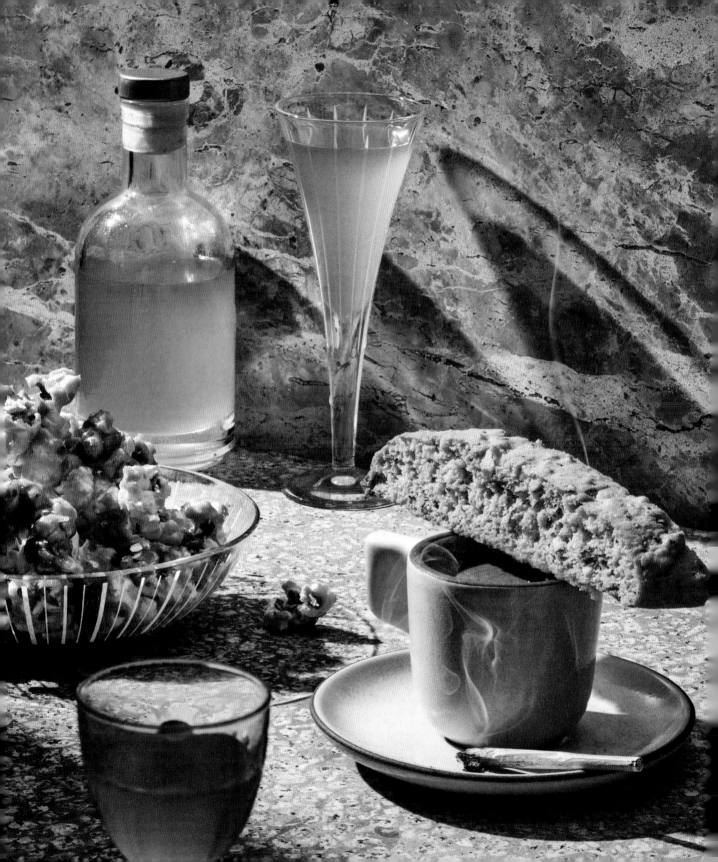

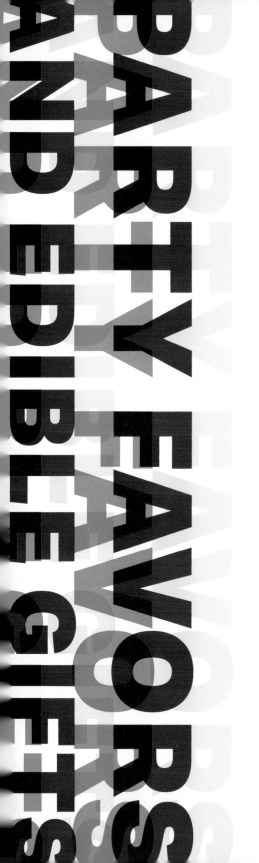

PARTY FAVORS
AND EDIBLE GIFTS

Send guests home on a high note with the ultimate goodie bags. These shelf-stable pot-presents let friends partake from the comfort of their own beds (or baths or couches). From buttery balms to lit liqueurs, give the gift of THC and everyone will RSVP yes for your parties.

CRACKER JANE

SERVES 8

TIME: 45 minutes

DOSE: 6.25 mg THC
per cup of popcorn

Meet Cracker Jane, the stoner Canadian cousin of the beloved American baseball game snack. While molasses builds the flavor for the classic treat, this rendition swaps the thick blackstrap for delicate maple syrup. Eat it by the handful, but with caution: The prize at the bottom of the box takes an hour to hit.

1 / Preheat the oven to 250°F.

2 / Grease a sheet pan and a large bowl and set both aside.

3 / Heat the oil in a large heavy-bottomed pot or Dutch oven over medium heat, then add 2 kernels of popcorn and cover. When both kernels pop, 2 to 3 minutes, remove the popped kernels and add the rest of the kernels to the pot. Replace the lid and turn the heat to medium-low. Gently shake the pot back and forth on the burner every 30 seconds, to ensure the popcorn heats evenly. The pops will get more frequent, then peak and start to slow down. Cook until you hear 3-second pauses in between pops, about 3 minutes. Transfer the popcorn to the prepared bowl and add the peanuts.

4 / In a 2-quart saucepan over medium-low heat, use a rubber spatula to stir together both butters, the sugar, maple syrup, and salt. Cook, stirring every minute until the caramel bubbles up and reaches 250°F, 8 to 10 minutes.

5 / Add the vanilla extract and baking soda and stir quickly as it bubbles up, then drizzle the caramel all over the popcorn and peanuts. Use an oven mitt to hold the bowl with one hand and the spatula in the other and stir. Scoop from the bottom and make sure to coat each kernel in the sticky sauce.

6 / Spread the popcorn out evenly on the prepared sheet pan and bake for 13 to 15 minutes, until the candy becomes brittle, rather than tacky. Once cooled, it should feel crisp. If it still feels sticky after removing from the oven, pop the pan back in the oven for another minute or two.

2 tablespoons neutral oil such as vegetable or canola, plus more for greasing

1/3 cup popcorn kernels

1/2 cup roasted, salted red-skin peanuts

1/2 cup (4 ounces) unsalted butter

2 tablespoons (1 ounce) Cannabutter (page 61)

3/4 cup (150 grams) granulated sugar

1/4 cup maple syrup

1/2 teaspoon kosher salt

1 teaspoon vanilla extract

1/4 teaspoon baking soda

HEADS UP, POTHEAD!
To give this snackable treat as a gift, go to your local craft store or online and pick up cellophane bags, labels, and some ribbon (I prefer grosgrain) to tie a bow on these dignified dime bags.

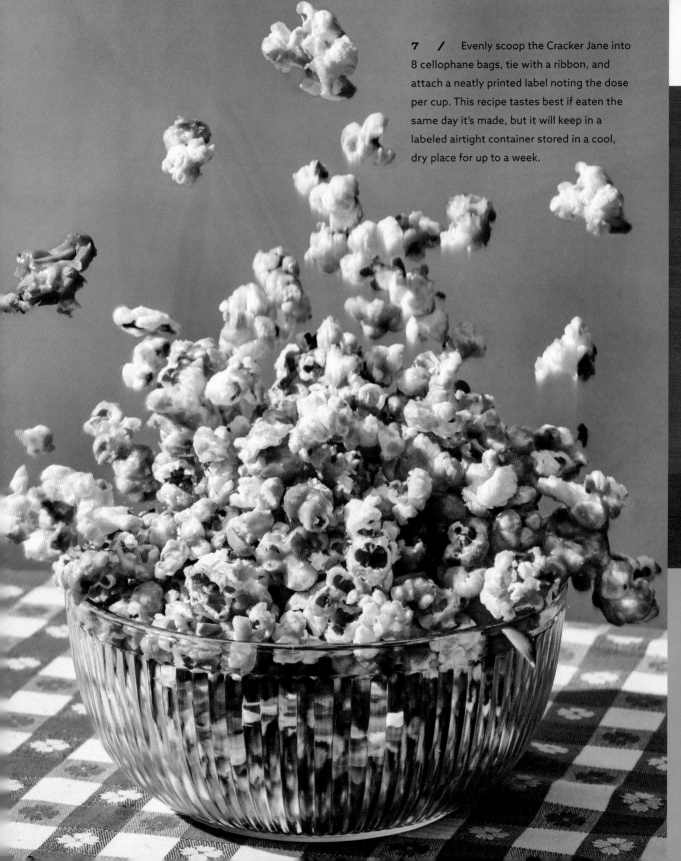

7 / Evenly scoop the Cracker Jane into 8 cellophane bags, tie with a ribbon, and attach a neatly printed label noting the dose per cup. This recipe tastes best if eaten the same day it's made, but it will keep in a labeled airtight container stored in a cool, dry place for up to a week.

FADED SUNDAE FUDGE SAUCE

MAKES 2 cups

TIME: 40 minutes

DOSE: 12.5 mg THC per ¼ cup

HEADS UP, POTHEAD!

If you plan to give this as a gift, have four 4-ounce glass jars with lids on hand.

Presumably my ex meant well when he offered to deliver forty boxes of chocolates from my house in San Francisco to my client in Los Angeles, but six hours in the back of his Prius in California's summer heat turned the pristine hash caramels into highly potent puddles.

I couldn't fathom throwing away the melted cannabis confections, so I scooped the goop from the bottom of each candy cup into a pot. I added a bunch of cream, a cup of cocoa powder, gave it a good whisk, and voilà: hot fudge sauce—which I jarred and sold, and which inspired this recipe. Thick enough to coat the back of a spoon, this fudge sauce makes getting high easy like an ice cream sundae.

1 / In a small saucepan set over low heat, whisk together the half-and-half and salt, then keep warm over low heat while preparing the caramel.

2 / In a separate medium saucepan, warm the sugar over medium heat, stirring until it melts and caramelizes to a dark amber, about 5 minutes. Turn the heat to low and slowly add the half-and-half to the sugar, watching carefully, as it will bubble up. Whisk the sauce until the caramel fully dissolves, about 3 minutes, then remove from the heat. Sift in the cocoa powder and whisk in the cannabutter and chocolate chips. When the chocolate fully melts, add the vanilla extract and give it a final vigorous whisk to combine. Pour the finished sauce through a mesh strainer to remove any lumps and let cool. Refrigerate in a labeled airtight container for up to 2 weeks.

3 / To jar the sauce as a gift, boil four 4-ounce glass jars and their lids in a large pot of water for 15 minutes. After removing from the water, flip the jars upside down to dry for a few minutes. Turn right-side up and fill with the hot fudge sauce, leaving a half-inch gap at the top. Twist on the sterilized lids and then circle back to tighten them. Boil the filled, sealed jars again for 5 minutes, then let cool on a towel. Tighten the lid one more time after they are fully cooled, if necessary. Label the jars of fudge sauce with the dose and to store in the fridge for up to 2 months.

2 cups half-and-half

½ teaspoon fine sea salt

1 cup (200 grams) granulated sugar

1 cup (90 grams) Dutch-process cocoa powder

⅓ cup (2⅔ ounce) Brown Cannabutter (page 62)

⅓ cup (2 ounces) bittersweet chocolate chips

½ teaspoon vanilla extract

SERVING SUGGESTION: Serve over ice cream, blend a scoopful into a Chilled-Out Almond Mocha (page 150), or put in jars to give this dosed delight away to friends by following the instructions after the recipe.

INTERSTELLAR STRAWBERRY JAM

MAKES 2½ cups

TIME: 45 minutes

DOSE: 1.5 mg THC per tablespoon of jam

During peak strawberry season when I lived in San Francisco, I often walked down Guerrero to the original Tartine Bakery, the one without a sign, and waited in line to buy a big buttery croissant with their house jam. I sat in Dolores Park and tore pieces of croissant apart, dipping it into the barely set jam.

Liz Prueitt, Tartine's founder, shopped at the chic clothing store I worked at in Hayes Valley. One day, as I gushed about her jam while pinning her dress for the James Beard awards (a floral Dries Van Noten number), she offered to teach me how to make that extraordinary jam. We became friends as she explained her general ratio of 3:1 fruit to sugar (by weight) and how to watch for the snap of the bubbles as the jam begins to gel. Liz skipped the (canna)butter in her recipe, but many seasoned jam-makers add a knob or two to their pots to hinder foam.

1 / In a 3-quart saucepan, sprinkle the sugar over the strawberries. Use a rubber spatula to stir them together, then set the pot over medium heat. Add the cannabutter, lemon juice, vanilla extract, lemon zest, and salt. Stir occasionally in the beginning, then constantly once the bubbles get large and plop when they pop. Remove from the heat when the temperature reaches 215°F, 30 to 35 minutes.

2 / If you are canning the jam, fill a large pot with water and boil over medium heat. Sterilize the jars by boiling for 10 minutes and letting dry upside down on a towel. Pour the jam into the prepared, sterilized jars, tighten the lids, and boil for 5 minutes. Let cool upside down. When fully cool, about 2 hours, label clearly with the dose, date, and a recommendation to store in the refrigerator and eat within a month. If you are not canning it, let the jam fully cool, then store in a labeled airtight container (or containers) in the refrigerator for up to 2 weeks.

1 cup (200 grams) granulated sugar

4 cups cored and quartered strawberries (about 1½ pounds)

2 tablespoons (1 ounce) Cannabutter (page 61)

2 tablespoons freshly squeezed lemon juice (about ½ a lemon)

1 tablespoon vanilla extract

½ tablespoon grated lemon zest (about 1 lemon)

¼ teaspoon fine sea salt

HEADS UP, POTHEAD!
If you plan to can this jam, have four 4-ounce glass jars ready to sterilize.

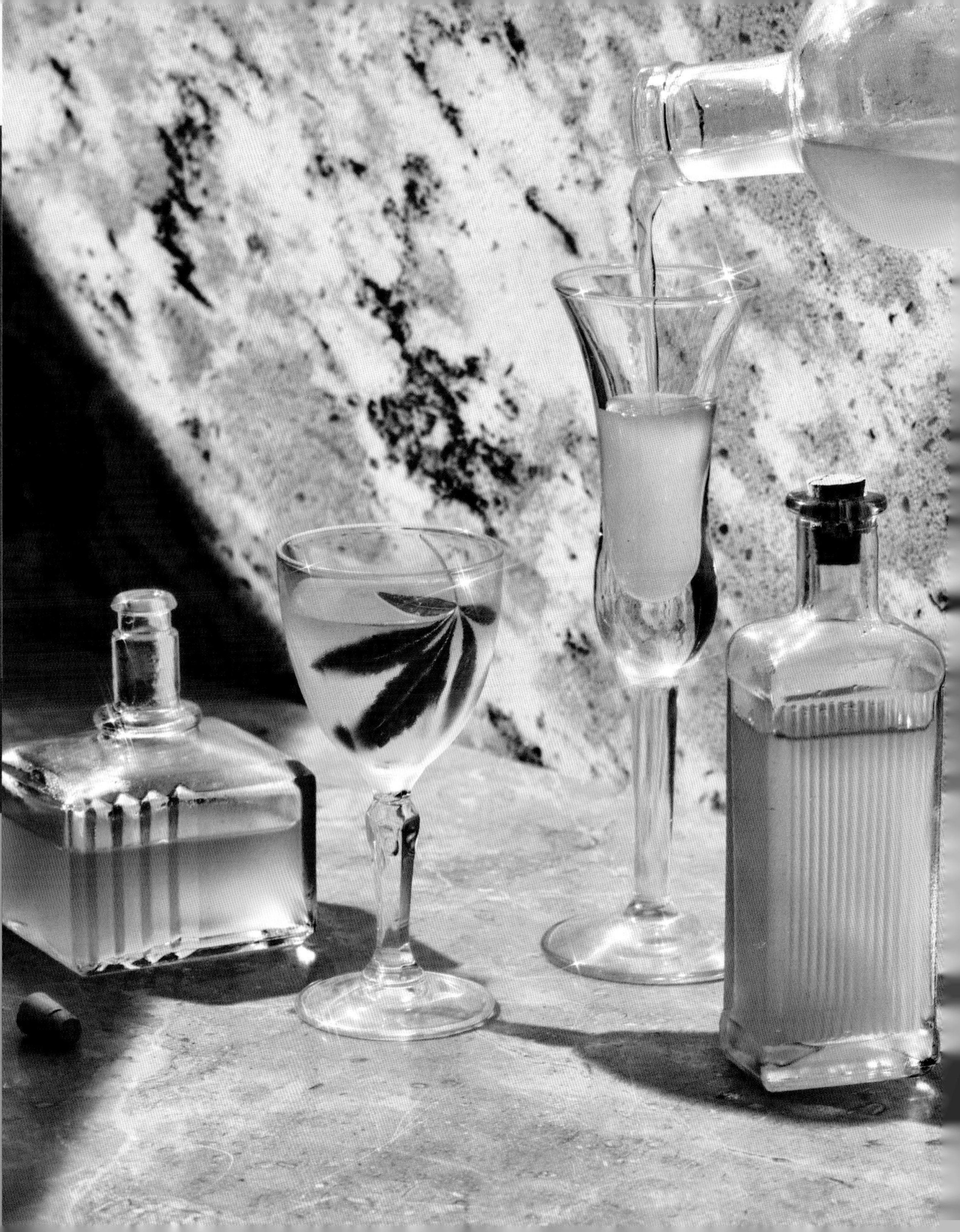

LIT LIMONCELLO

MAKES 6 (200 ml) bottles

TIME: 1 month

DOSE: 2.5 mg THC per 50 ml shot

When life gives you lemons, make weed-infused limoncello. While I shy away from crossfading, only a fool gets wasted on limoncello. Drizzle it over ice cream, soak it into a coffee cake, or simply sip cold from a glass: This limoncello bottles the bright flavor of lemons alongside the potent effects of weed.

The higher the proof of your starting spirit, the less time the lemon peel needs to sit in the liquor to extract all the limonene (the main terpene found in citrus, which imparts flavor and aroma). Avoid the shiny conventional lemons at the grocery store, since they get coated in a wax that hinders the alcohol from reaching the peel; organic or homegrown lemons work best.

1 / Use a vegetable peeler to remove the yellow peel from all the lemons. Use a paring knife to remove any remaining pith on the peels, as this will impart a bitter flavor to the limoncello.

2 / Place the lemon peels in a clean, dry, 32-ounce glass jar. Pour the entire bottle of alcohol over the peels, screw on the lid, and give it a gentle shake. Store the jar in a cool dark place for 2 to 3 weeks, shaking for a few seconds every other day.

3 / Taste the infusion starting after 2 weeks to check for a bright, potent lemon flavor. When it has an intense citrus flavor and yellow color, strain the liquor into a large bowl.

4 / Finish the process by making the simple syrup: In a 2-quart saucepan over medium heat, whisk together the sugar and water until the sugar dissolves, 2 to 3 minutes. Let cool completely before adding it to the lemon liqueur and whisking in the Turnt Tincture.

5 / Line up 6 bottles, 200 milliliters each, and use a funnel and ladle to fill with the infused limoncello.

6 / Limoncello tastes best when it sits and the alcohol mellows for an additional month but can be sipped immediately. Label clearly with the dose and gift to friends who imbibe.

8 to 10 organic lemons

1 (750 ml) bottle 120-proof neutral alcohol, such as Everclear

2 cups (400 grams) granulated sugar

1 cup water

2 tablespoons Freezer Turnt Tincture (page 70)

HEADS UP, POTHEAD!
To bottle the limoncello, have six 200-milliliter bottles sterilized and ready.

ROSEMARY-JANE BISCOTTI

MAKES 24 biscotti

TIME: 1 hour 30 minutes

DOSE: 4 mg THC per biscotti

At a friend's Italian Sunday supper, the host plopped down a Prada tie box on the table. We opened it to reveal dozens of identically sliced and evenly baked rosemary biscotti, each speckled with nuts and made that morning by his Calabrian mother. I baptized the first one in vin santo, took a bite, and knew immediately that I had to have the recipe. Luckily, my friend's mom doesn't believe in recipe gatekeeping, and neither do I.

1 / Preheat the oven to 350°F. Line a sheet pan with parchment paper.

2 / Spread the almonds over the sheet pan and bake for 5 to 6 minutes, until they smell toasty but haven't yet browned. Transfer to a small bowl and set aside to cool. Keep the sheet pan with the parchment paper ready.

3 / In a medium bowl, whisk together the flour, baking powder, and salt. In a separate large bowl, use a handheld mixer on medium speed to beat the cannabutter, unsalted butter, and sugar to a light, creamy consistency, 1 to 2 minutes. Then add the eggs, one at a time, mixing until each is fully incorporated, and, after the second, until the mixture turns a pale yellow color, 2 to 3 minutes. The batter will break and the flour will bring it back together later. Add the rosemary, vanilla extract, and lemon zest and beat for another 15 seconds, just to incorporate the aromatics. With a large rubber spatula, fold in the dry ingredients. When just a few streaks of flour remain in the batter, add the toasted almonds and give the mixture a few final turns to distribute the nuts and mix in the last of the flour. Avoid overmixing, as the biscotti will get tough. The dough will be soft like frosting; that's okay. Do not add more flour.

¾ cup (95 grams) roughly chopped raw almonds

1½ cups (180 grams) all-purpose flour

2 teaspoons baking powder

½ teaspoon kosher salt

¼ cup (2 ounces) Cannabutter (page 61), room temperature

¼ cup (2 ounces) unsalted butter, room temperature

½ cup (100 grams) granulated sugar

2 large eggs

2 tablespoons chopped fresh rosemary

1½ teaspoons vanilla extract

1 teaspoon grated lemon zest (about ½ a large lemon)

recipe continues

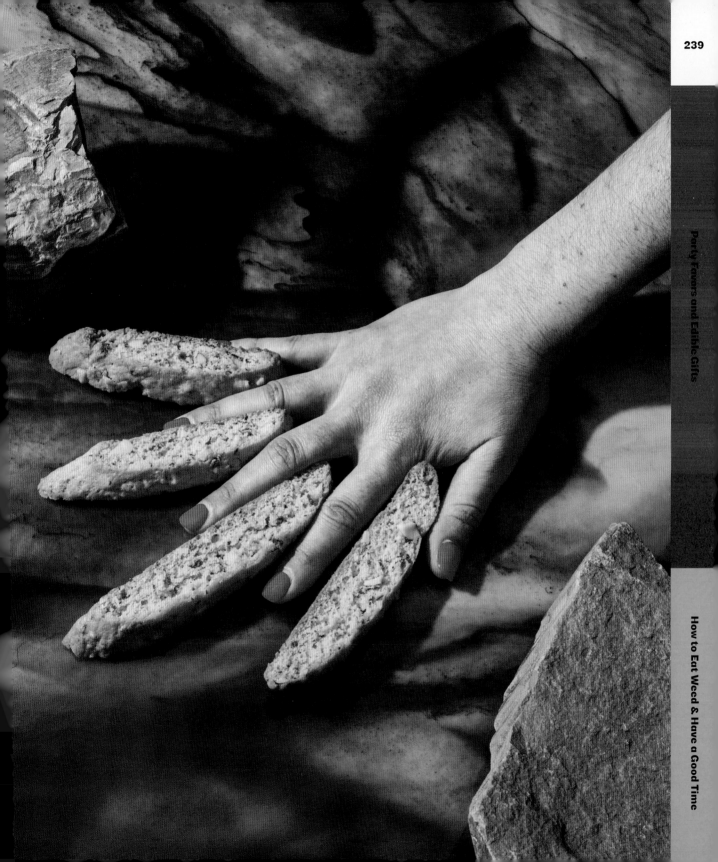

4 / Scoop half of the dough onto the prepared sheet pan and use the spatula to shape it into a rectangle 3 inches wide, 9½ inches long, and 1 inch tall. Repeat with the second half of the dough. Pop the sheet pan in the fridge for 15 minutes, to avoid overspreading, then bake the logs for 20 to 22 minutes, until the bottoms turn honey gold but the tops stay pale. Let cool on the pan for 5 minutes. Turn the oven down to 325°F.

5 / Use a very sharp knife to slice the logs on a long diagonal into two dozen ¾-inch-thick cookies. I eat the short diagonal nubbins on the end. Place the cookies cut side down on the sheet pan. Bake for 10 minutes, then flip the cookies and bake for another 8 minutes. Remove from the oven and let cool fully on a wire rack.

6 / Serve right away or package in cellophane bags, tie with a string, and attach a label with the dose.

SERVING SUGGESTION: Give the gift of la dolce vita with these and a bottle of Lit Limoncello (page 237).

POT COCOA MIX

MAKES 6 (1-cup) bags or jars

TIME: 10 minutes

DOSE: 3.5 mg THC per ¼ cup of mix

We all need a sippable, discreet way to get high around family. This instant-cocoa-with-a-kick stirs into a cup of hot water and lasts long enough to get through the bulk of the holidays. The Dutch-process cocoa gives this infused mix an extra chocolatey punch, and the custard powder thickens the drink into an irresistibly rich and silky brew.

1 / In a food processor, pulse together all of the ingredients a few times, until evenly blended. Divide the mix among 6 zip-top bags.

2 / Seal and store in a cool, dry place for up to 2 months. For extra-fancy hot cocoa gifts, put the bag in a metal tin or fun coffee mug, or package the mix in 8-ounce mason jars.

3 / Write the following preparation instructions on an attached card: "To prepare cocoa: Stir together ¼ cup of mix and 1 cup of hot water until completely dissolved."

2 cups (200 grams) nonfat dry milk powder

2 cups (180 grams) unsweetened Dutch-process cocoa powder

1 cup (200 grams) granulated sugar

1 cup (200 grams) dark brown sugar

½ cup (100 grams) Stoned Sugar (page 77)

½ cup (80 grams) custard powder (such as Bird's)

1 teaspoon kosher salt

SERVING SUGGESTION: Wrap it up with one or two Marshmellows (page 215).

LOVE THYSELF LAVENDER BATH SALTS

MAKES 6
(8-ounce) jars

TIME: 40 minutes

DOSE: 100 mg THC
per jar

Self-care goddess Angela Lansbury called taking a relaxing bath a "great ceremony." Cleopatra bathed in milk and Marilyn Monroe took a dip in Champagne, but I recommend tapping into the anti-inflammatory benefits of weed for a soothing soak. Since our skin cells contain endocannabinoid receptors, THC helps Epsom salts melt away achy muscles and reduce inflammation. The skin also acts as a barrier, preventing topical cannabinoids from reaching the bloodstream, so I maximize the THC to optimize the benefits. The effects remain localized, making these a thoughtful gift to friends who abstain from the psychoactive effects of THC but still need a little TLC. Label the jar "Love Thyself Lavender Bath Salts (100 Milligrams THC)."

1 / Preheat the oven to 240°F.

2 / In an oven-safe bowl, bake the olive oil for about 10 minutes, until the temperature reaches 240°F. Use a spoon to stir the flower in for 30 seconds, then put the bowl back into the oven for 20 more minutes, stirring every 5 minutes. Pour the infused oil through a cheesecloth-lined strainer into a large bowl. Let cool for a few minutes before gathering the cheesecloth, squeezing out any excess oil, and discarding the flower.

3 / Use a rubber spatula to stir the Epsom salt, sea salt, dried lavender (if using), and lavender essential oil into the infused olive oil until thoroughly combined, about 2 minutes.

4 / Divide the salt evenly among the 6 jars and label with the amount of THC. Use within a year.

¼ cup extra-virgin olive oil

3 grams ground decarboxylated flower

4 cups Epsom salt

2 cups coarse sea salt

¼ cup dried lavender (optional)

½ teaspoon (50 drops) lavender essential oil

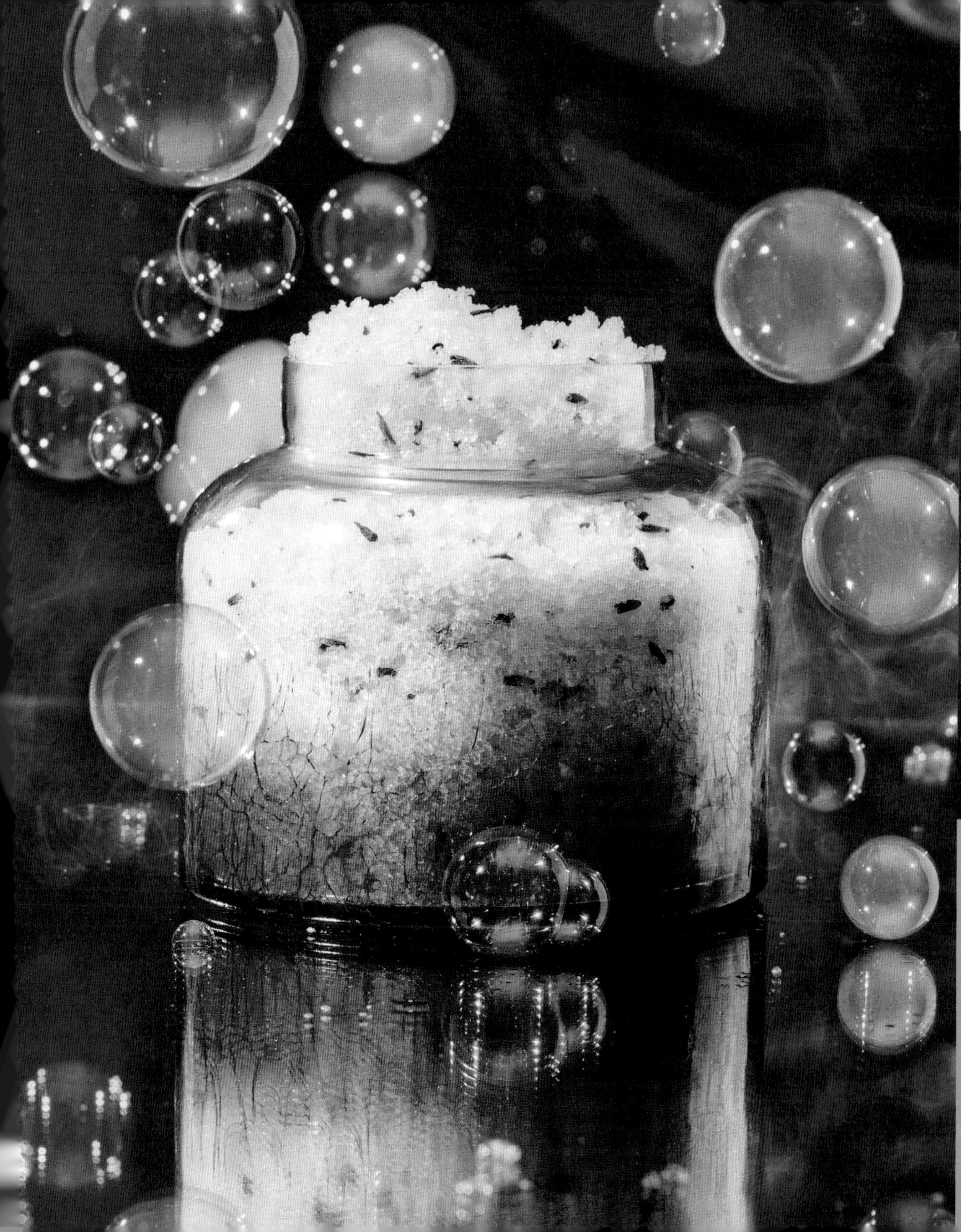

SAVIOR SALVE

MAKES 5
(4-ounce) jars

TIME: 20 minutes

DOSE: 120 mg THC
per jar

I wash a lot of dishes, I garden without gloves, and I lift heavy weights. To help my hands stay soft, I apply this infused balm before bed. The cannabis works alongside another therapeutic herb, known scientifically as *Arnica montana* and colloquially as mountain tobacco—although I've never smoked it. Together, the two herbs provide anti-inflammatory benefits, while the cooling menthol in the peppermint oil soothes skin. Whenever I visit my aunty Yo, we make a big batch using her trim and my uncle's beeswax. Before giving the jars as gifts, make sure to label each "Savior Salve: For topical use only" and the amount of THC in the jar.

1 / Fill a large pot with water, heat on medium-high, then boil five 4-ounce jars for 10 minutes to sterilize them. Remove and let dry upside down on a clean kitchen towel.

2 / Make a double boiler by filling a 3-quart saucepan with 2 cups of water and placing a medium metal bowl on top. Set the double boiler over medium-low heat. In the bowl, use a rubber spatula to stir together the coconut oil and beeswax. Once the beeswax fully melts, 5 to 6 minutes, remove the bowl from the saucepan.

3 / Stir in the shea butter, arnica oil, and peppermint oil, until the shea butter fully melts from the residual heat. Divide the blended salve evenly between the jars and let cool for an hour before screwing on the lids and labeling. The salve lasts for up to 6 months.

1½ cups OOO Coconut Oil (page 64)

½ cup chopped beeswax

½ cup shea butter

2 tablespoons arnica oil

1 tablespoon peppermint oil

ACKNOWLEDGMENTS

This book would never have been written without my collaborator Naomi Tomky. She took on this book and turned it into a comprehensive text. A huge amount of gratitude to her and her family for the time and mental gymnastics she provided.

Thank you to Justin Schwartz, my editor at Simon Element, who saw the potential in me and whose sharp eye helped shape this into a truly cookable book.

My agent, Kari Stuart, who stuck with me in every iteration of the proposal, will always have my gratitude.

Huge appreciation to the incredible team who brought the book visually to life: My photographer, Julia Stotz, who tapped into her inner stoner; her lighting tech, Sherman Lee, and his assistant, Briley; her second photo assistant, Brian Chism; our food stylist extraordinaire, Casey Dobbins, with assistants Courtney Weis and Max Rappaport; incredible set designer Samantha Margherita and assistant Ruth Kim; my wardrobe stylist, Ashley Guerzon, for dressing me like a posh pothead; and Janelle Detina, for the glam. Thank you to Nico Pisarro at Proplink Studios and Julia Tsao for her beautiful home. A special thank-you to illustrator Maria Schoettler, who painted watercolors of the cannabis plant and illustrated decarboxylation and the terpene chart.

A big thank-you to my dear friend Nina Gregory, who combed through every line, and Regina Castillo for copyediting. To Jen Wang, who laid out the design of this book, my eternal gratitude for bringing a fun flow and vibrant style to the pages.

Love to my aunty Yo for the recipes and inspiration; and to my uncle Ned, thank you for the macadamia nuts and jars of honey, and for always believing in me.

To my creative sounding board Eddy Moretti, who came up with the name for this book, *grazie mille*. A big thank-you to my testers who made sure all eighty infused recipes worked: Alexander Roberts, Amanda Berrill, Jen Shelbo, and Emily Tylman. And to artist Niki Ford, who got stoned with me and brainstormed punny recipe names.

I couldn't have conducted as many experiments as I did without the fresh flowers; thanks to Joaquin and Luis Bobadilla and Lauren McGonagle of Mota Los Angeles. I worked with two different labs to pinpoint the science behind this book: Thank you to Angie Macaraeg at Encore Labs and Sidney Cobos from Caligreen Laboratory.

To my modern family, Scott Goble, Ben Ospital, Chris Ospital, and Geri Ospital, thank you for always supporting me. And to Mary, for the wisdom and hash.

A lot of gratitude goes to my dog, BonBon, whom I adopted when I first started writing this book; she kept me walking every day, high as a kite.

GLOSSARY

ANTHOCYANIN: The water-soluble flavonoid pigment responsible for purple cauliflower, red berries, and violet weed, like Purple Kush.

BADDER: A sticky, terpene-rich, solvent-extracted cannabis concentrate that is whipped to a frosting texture.

BHANG: A paste made from cannabis leaves and flowers, used mostly in drinks and food in India, particularly during the holiday of Holi.

BLUNT: Cannabis wrapped in a hollowed-out cigar or other form of tobacco leaf, designed for smoking. Usually fat.

BONG: A water pipe, which cools the cannabis smoke, making it less harsh and allowing for bigger rips.

BOWL: The small circular receptacle that holds the weed in pipes, bubblers, and bongs.

BUD: Chunks of cannabis flower. Also, a general term for cannabis.

BUDDER: A terpene-rich, solvent-extracted cannabis concentrate made into a light wax using pressure and heat.

CANNABINOIDS: The compounds that give weed its potency, including the potentially psychoactive one, THCA.

CANNABIS: A genus of flowering plants with psychotropic effects on humans. Also known as weed.

CBD (CANNABIDIOL): A phytocannabinoid that is one of the active compounds in cannabis and has many therapeutic effects.

CBN (CANNABINOL): A compound resulting from the degradation of THC in weed that has soporific effects; possibly to blame for your couch lock.

CHERRY: The glow of a still-lit bowl or joint, which means if you're not inhaling, weed is going to waste.

COLA: The largest bud at the top of the cannabis plant or any cluster of flowers growing tightly together on a stem.

CONCENTRATES: Refined forms of cannabis that hyper-concentrate the best parts of the weed into the smallest volumes.

CULTIVAR: A specific variety of weed, distinguished by plant genetics and how it looks, smells, or affects the user.

DABS: Cannabis concentrates inhaled by vaporization.

DISTILLATE: A tasteless, decarboxylated form of liquid cannabis concentrate with all plant matter, terpenes, and flavonoids removed, leaving only cannabinoids.

EDIBLES: Food, but with weed in it.

ENDOCANNABINOID SYSTEM: A collection of receptors for cannabinoids all over our bodies that regulates a majority of our bodily functions, including appetite and anxiety.

FLAVONOIDS: Flavor compounds responsible for the taste of various weed strains.

FLOWER: The part of the plant with all the power—the trichome-laden bud of the female cannabis plant.

GRINDER: A tool designed to break up cannabis into small pieces ideal for cooking with (or smoking).

HASH: A raw concentrate made by compressing cannabis, specifically the resin-heavy parts, into a brick or ball.

HASH OIL: A highly potent solvent-extracted cannabis concentrate and the base for many terpene-rich concentrates.

HASH ROSIN: A solventless cannabis concentrate made by pressing and heating hash.

HEMP: Cannabis cultivated specifically for lower THC levels, for use in therapeutics, fibers, and other typically non-psychoactive applications.

INDICA: Shorter, faster-growing cannabis strains with more buds, thought to give more of a body high.

JOINT: A cannabis cigarette.

KIEF: Collected concentrated cannabis crystals or trichomes (sometimes with small plant fragments).

LIVE RESIN: A cannabis concentrate made from solvent-extracted fresh-frozen cannabis plants.

LIVE ROSIN: A solventless cannabis concentrate made from pressed fresh-frozen cannabis plants.

POTENCY: The THC percentage of any given flower, edible, or concentrate.

SATIVA: Strains of cannabis that grow taller, with longer fan leaves. Thought to give a more cerebral, upbeat, zippy high.

SHAKE: The loose bits of plant matter that break off from the bud during handling or processing.

SHATTER: A solid, translucent, and terpene-rich cannabis concentrate, named for its glass-like appearance.

STRAIN: See *cultivar*.

SUGAR LEAF: The small, trichome covered leaves that grow in cannabis flowers and get trimmed off in processing.

TINCTURE: A type of cannabis extract made by soaking the flower in alcohol.

TERPENE: The compound that makes essential oils—and cannabis—smell the way they do.

TOPICAL: Cannabis products applied externally, like salves or lotions.

TRICHOME: The small glandular hairs that concentrate on cannabis flowers and secrete the resin that contains the cannabinoids.

TRIM: The pieces of sugar leaf removed in the harvesting and processing of the cannabis plant, usually with lower potency than full buds.

WAX: A category of terpene-rich cannabis concentrates named for their texture.

Glossary

How to Eat Weed & Have a Good Time

INDEX

Index

SIMON
ELEMENT

An Imprint of Simon & Schuster, LLC
1230 Avenue of the Americas
New York, NY 10020

First Simon Element hardcover edition
April 2025

SIMON ELEMENT is a trademark of Simon &
Schuster, LLC

For information about special discounts for
bulk purchases, please contact Simon &
Schuster Special Sales at 1-866-506-1949 or
business@simonandschuster.com.

The Simon & Schuster Speakers Bureau can
bring authors to your live event. For more
information or to book an event, contact the
Simon & Schuster Speakers Bureau at
1-866-248-3049 or visit our website at
www.simonspeakers.com.

Interior design by Jen Wang

Food styling by Casey Dobbins

Prop styling by Samantha Margherita

Manufactured in China

10 9 8 7 6 5 4 3 2 1

Library of Congress Cataloging-in-Publication
Data has been applied for.

ISBN 978-1-6680-4929-7
ISBN 978-1-6680-4930-3 (ebook)